Masaki Nishina

Edited by Amanda Jayne

# Reiki and Japan

## A Cultural View of Western and Japanese Reiki

2017-A edition

The information in this book has been carefully researched and presented to the best of the author's knowledge and consciousness. Despite this fact, neither the author nor publisher assume any type of liability for presumed or actual damages of any kind that might result from the direct or indirect application of the statements in this book.

# Table of Contents

## Preface

This book is an account of Japanese Reiki. It looks at the effects of Japanese history, particularly the prewar and postwar periods, on Reiki and other alternative therapies. It also details the extent to which cultural backgrounds have made Japanese and Western Reiki different.

I wrote my first Reiki book in 2009 and dedicated one chapter to the historical background of Reiki, but it was omitted from the final manuscript because the publisher did not think the general public would be interested. For me, however, learning about the history of both Japanese and Western Reiki, and studying their similarities and differences, has been fascinating. I published a book on this in Japanese in 2013 and am now very happy to provide an English edition of that book.

Reiki therapy was born in 1920s Japan and thrived until the postwar occupation of Japan brought catastrophic changes that had a radical effect on the way people lived and thought. The use of traditional therapies, including Reiki, rapidly declined as a result. Eventually, 'new' methods, including Western Reiki, were imported from abroad. The more I learned of Japanese history, the more I recognized the many precious treasures Japanese culture has to offer, treasures that are forgotten, ignored or have been lost.

This book answers the following questions:

- Why was Reiki born in Japan?

- How did people use Reiki before the war?

- Were there any other therapies like Reiki at that time?

- Why did people stop using Reiki after the war in Japan?

- What exactly is Western Reiki?

- How different is Western Reiki from Japanese Reiki?

- Why Western Reiki and Japanese Reiki are different?

- Why did Western practitioners invent the master symbol?

These are interesting questions, yet to date, few books have been available to answer them.

I have also intended that this book helps people understand what Reiki really is and enhance readers' daily Reiki practices. It is written with the assumption that readers are already familiar with Reiki, especially Western Reiki. Anyone can start using Reiki without knowing its history. However one can only understand the most important aspects of Reiki by knowing the historical details and understanding the cultural background it came from. These are not taught in Reiki seminars. Though the content of this book is not essentially for Reiki beginners, anyone who reads and understands it should be able to practice Reiki more smoothly with a higher awareness.

This book is unique in its detailed comparison between Japanese Reiki and Western Reiki. Very few books do this, probably because few Reiki teachers have enough experience teaching both to fully grasp the necessary details.

There are a huge number of Reiki publications available in the Western market, but there are only a few pieces of literature that can truly be trusted. I have listed them below.

1. *Reiki Therapy Handbook* (霊気療法のしおり) edited by Usui Reiki Ryoho Gakkai in 1974.

This is very precious. It is first-class literature but has not been published commercially and has no English translation at this time. It is a 'must read' if anyone wants to understand Japanese Reiki. *Reiki Therapy Handbook* describes some historical facts as well, but because of copyright, it is not available in the West.

2. *Jikiden Reiki* written by Tadao Yamaguchi and first published in English in 2007 under the name, *Light on the Origins of Reiki* (ISBN: 0914955659). The author of this book has been practicing Japanese Reiki all his life. He learned with his mother, who learned Reiki from Chujiro Hayashi. They collected the historical information and photographs from their relatives who also learned Reiki from Hayashi before the war.

The authors of these two books actually practiced Japanese Reiki free from the influence of postwar Western culture in Japan, making them more trustworthy

3. *This is Reiki* written by Frank Arjava Petter in 2012 (ISBN: 0940985012). This book provides the most complete historical information on Reiki

available. The author visited the historical places he mentions and met the relevant people.

4. *The Hayashi Reiki Manual* written by Frank Arjava Petter and Tadao Yamaguchi in 2003 (ISBN: 0914955756).
This book provides a great deal of historical information on Reiki and contains some precious photographs.

5. *Reiki: Iyashino-te* written by Toshitaka Mochizuki, (Kindle edition ASIN: B01KWJ9XI8).
Due to the fact that the author became acquainted with some members of the Usui Reiki Ryoho Gakkai, this book provides important historical information and contains precious photographs. However, please note that the manga part of this book contains false information on Master Usui, adversely affected by Western Reiki.

6. *Reiki, Energy Filling the Universe* (レイキ 宇宙に満ちるエネルギー) written by Hiroshi Doi in 2005 (Japanese edition only ISBN: 4861060338). The author is a member of the Usui Reiki Ryoho Gakkai and this book contains important historical information that he obtained there.

Readers should know that books not listed here may carry false information. Authors of literature on Western Reiki especially, tend to copy historical information from existing Western Reiki books without confirming their accuracy. In addition, the information on the internet often contains a great many misunderstandings and distortions. I don't recommend you use this method to find accurate information.

While translating this book into English, I came to appreciate the extent of the language barrier between Japanese and other Western languages. There are actually many good books on Japanese history and culture but unfortunately most of them remain unpublished in Western languages. Japanese people are generally not interested in promoting information about themselves abroad.

In this book, when I describe the Japanese history related to Japanese and Western Reiki, it is based on various items of literature I have studied and of course is embedded with my world view and historical understanding. It is still possible that I have misunderstood something or found information that proves to be false. If that is the case, I would be very happy to hear from readers.

With love and gratitude,
Masaki Nishina
Spring, 2017

## Foreword

### by Amanda Jayne

I first learned Reiki in 2002 with Chiyoko Yamaguchi in her small Kyoto home. She was very welcoming and open to teaching me, a Westerner, the precious Reiki she had learned so long ago. As I attended more classes, I met other Westerners who had flown to Japan to learn from Chiyoko Yamaguchi and her son Tadao. I began to see just how differently Westerners were looking at Reiki and noticed how often Chiyoko Yamaguchi was surprised or confused by the questions they asked. "You think too much," she would say to us with a smile. It's true, I did. I probably still do. The cultures she and I came from are oceans apart in so many ways. I spent five years living in Japan and the longer I lived there, the less I understood the culture. I had imagined that after one or two years, I'd really have it down and 'get' the Japanese and their way of life. Little did I know! By the time I left in 2006, I had learned a great deal and begun to understand a little about the different ways Japanese and Westerners approach life, but it wasn't until I came across Masaki Nishina's work that I started to understand why it was so difficult to understand.

The truth is, the Japanese culture has been remarkably flexible in allowing aspects of other cultures to join it quite harmoniously, like tributaries flowing into a main stem river. It makes for a wonderful cacophony of old and new, East and West, that is delightful to visiting tourists and highly confusing to non-Japanese who live there and try to understand what's really going on. What Masaki is so clear on, is how vitally important it is that the unique aspects of the ancient Japanese culture are not lost. Modern

13

Japanese, he says, are losing connection with their ancient roots and what those roots have to teach us about life and living are essential to all our futures.

What does this have to do with Reiki? Everything. As Masaki explains in this book, understanding the original Japanese culture is the only way to truly understand what Reiki really is. He takes us on a journey to help us all comprehend not only the truth about the natural simplicity of Reiki energy, but also the fascinating historical, social and political climate into which Reiki therapy emerged.

Masaki's research is valuable to anyone interested in Reiki. As I have worked with him, I have come to respect him greatly and admire his integrity when dealing with historical information. I have come to see he is not just interested in finding information to fit in with what he believes, he wants to provide facts and present what really happened to the best of his ability. Likewise, he does not take sides when looking at different types of Reiki. There are things he is critical of, but only in terms of finding the truth and helping people to see more of themselves. He sees the good in both Eastern and Western cultures.

I have found that reading and editing this book has brought me valuable insight into what happened to Reiki and why it changed so much as it travelled across the world. It has given me a new depth of appreciation of those who carried this incredible natural healing therapy through difficult times, doing all they could to make sure it was not lost. It has also brought me back to nature, to the roots of life itself, to Reiki.

I hope it does the same for you.

With love

Amanda Jayne

Jikiden Reiki Dai-shihan

Author, Editor, Illustrator

MA Spiritual Psychology

# Chapter 1  Reiki's Native Land

To understand anything thoroughly, it is vital to look at the environment from which it emerged. Reiki has travelled across the world and the Japanese soil that first germinated the seed has often been either forgotten or misunderstood. I hope to offer you more insight into the culture and environment that gave birth to Reiki.

## Japanese history

When *Mikao Usui* started Reiki in 1922, Japan was undergoing a period of significant change. During the late 19th and early 20th century, the Meiji period, the country began to establish the foundations of its modern structure. These changes inadvertently led to an increase in a variety of healing therapies. Let's look at the history and environment that caused the upsurge of so many therapies.

In Japan, the reign of each Emperor is given a name.

- Meiji (明治) era: 1868 - 1912
- Taisho (大正) era: 1912 - 1926
- Showa (昭和) era: 1926 - 1989
- Heisei (平成) era: 1989 - present day

When Japanese refer to a particular year, they use the name of the era and count from the start of that reign. So if Usui founded Reiki in 1922 in the

Western-used calendar, in the Japanese calendar it would have been Taisho 11.

The *Meiji Restoration* took place at the beginning of the Meiji period, around 1870. Until then, Japan had been governed by the Edo (江戸) shogunate and remained isolated from other countries for 300 years. In order to modernize the nation, the Meiji government enforced a top-down restoration and introduced Western values to Japan, leaving some traditional values behind. Anything Western was thought to be superior and more advanced leading Japanese people to lose confidence in their own traditional culture and values. This was the first experience of Japanese rejecting their own culture. This collective self-denial was later to happen in the extreme during the American occupation, but the Meiji Restoration brought about the first glimmer of a negative mindset that remains embedded in people's minds today.

While studying Reiki history, I have learned about the preciousness of Japanese culture fostered since ancient times. I have also come to see the importance of healing the erroneous view of our own culture.

**The rise of the military**
Japanese victory in the Russo-Japanese war (1904-1905) temporarily strengthened the military voice in Japan. However, it soon decreased again as a result of the Washington Naval Treaty in 1921 as the treaty placed strict limits on naval construction.

Around this time, people began talking openly about democracy and a greater liberalism began to creep into many aspects of society. In 1925 laws were changed so that all men could vote where previously only rich men were eligible. This era later became known as the *Taisho democracy*. However, not everything during this period heralded democracy. The government also passed a *Maintenance of Public Order* law that was said to be an important act to prevent terrorism, including communism. In practice, it suppressed any activity thought to be anti-government or anti-military and led to severe punishments for those said to be involved. This was simply a foreshadowing of the constraints that were to come.

In 1930 the London Naval Treaty imposed even stricter limits on naval construction. The Japanese Army grew angry at the restrictions and declared the treaty to be against the Emperor's will, eventually renouncing the treaty. At the same time, some were encouraging military action abroad in the name of globalization and to compensate for the economic issues created by the worldwide depression.

The wheel of destruction started to spin rapidly as the Army grew more powerful and refused to be controlled by the now weak government. In 1931 they carried out what's known as the *Manchurian Incident* of their own accord, laying explosives by a railway and accusing Chinese dissidents of the attack. This gave the Japanese Army an excuse to invade and led to their occupation of Manchuria. As a result, Japan withdrew from the League of Nations in 1933 and the Army continued their display of power by entering the second Sino-Japanese war in 1937. At home, the military were now starting to control many aspects of people's lives, influencing the government to pass the National Mobilization Law of 1938 that limited civil rights in Japan. The war against the US was initiated by the Navy's attack on Pearl Harbor in 1941. It is this period of around fifteen years, 1930-1945, that could be considered a dark period in Japanese history. I will discuss this further in Chapter 7.

## Prewar Japan - It's not all dark!

Since the defeat of World War II and the following occupation, the Japanese prewar history taught in schools has not been accurate. This was largely a result of propaganda and education policies brought about during the American occupation (as discussed in Chapter 8). Japanese students have long been given the impression that there was nothing good about prewar Japan. Some are taught of the militarism and totalitarianism that did happen for a period of time, but they are given the mistaken impression that it prevailed throughout the prewar eras from the Meiji period (1868) onward (Junji Banno and Souichiro Tahara *Democracy in Imperial Japan* ISBN 4093892423). I was never taught the many positive things that came out of prewar Japan either and, until recently, thought of it all as the dark ages.

In fact, it was during the Meiji to early Showa eras that Japan laid strong foundations for key components of present-day Japan. Many world-famous companies were founded in the Meiji era for example. A study by Tokyo Business & Industry Research indicates there are 7,441 long-established Japanese companies, of which 79% were founded during the Meiji era. Of 3,566 companies publicly listed on the stock exchange, 469 are more than

100 years old, born of these so-called dark ages. Many of these are household names today. For example, Toshiba (1904), Nissan (1911), Nikon (1917), Panasonic (1918) and Toyota (1933).

In addition to the industrial and economic importance of these eras, they also brought about some positive social and educational changes. Most major universities started in the early Meiji era and a great many elementary schools were built. The foundations of our modern school infrastructure were laid during this period.

I really feel excited looking at the history of these companies, universities and schools. Even though the Meiji Restoration encouraged people to leave traditional Japanese values behind and adapt to Western culture, we can't forget that it brought about the building of a new modern Japan. There is healthy and positive energy in this and it is not appropriate to dismiss it all as a dark age. The human connections and company organizations started in these prewar eras flow through to the present day and it was in this environment that Reiki first bloomed.

Anyone interested in learning more accurate information about Japanese history in the Meiji, Taisho and early Showa eras should read the following books:
  • Masahiko Fujiwara's *Dignity of the State* (2005)
    - ISBN 4896845684 (available in English and Japanese)
It is only recently that people have been able to freely publish books documenting the true history of Japan in these eras. Before then, it was

taboo to publish such books. These recent books are yet to be translated into foreign languages:

- Kazutoshi Hando's *Showa History* 1926-1945 (2006)
  - ISBN 4582766714 (Japanese edition only)
- Masahiko Fujiwara's *Japanese Pride* (2011)
  - ISBN 4166608045 (Japanese edition only)
- Satoko Akio's *Washington Heights* (2011)
  - ISBN 4101359865 (Japanese edition only)

## The strength in Japanese culture

Japan is the oldest country in the world. Its rich history and precious culture spans nearly 2,000 years [Source: Tsuneyasu Takeda *Why do Japanese not know Japan?* ISBN 4569799337]. Japan has remained a unified nation and has not faced outright civil war despite facing several significant periods in which the country and culture have been threatened.

The first is probably the *Taika Reforms* of 645 when the government of the time introduced various aspects of Chinese society including Buddhism into the culture. Gradually, rather than fighting it, people began to incorporate Buddhism into the native religious-like culture of *Shinto* (神道, the way of God). I talk more about Shinto in Chapters 11 and 13.

A second example is the Meiji Restoration after the fall of the Edo shogunate. The new government, partly in preparation to defend against any attempt at colonization by Western countries, began a period of modernization and brought in some aspects of Western culture and ideas.

At this time, an astounding event took place that illustrates the ability of Japanese to adapt, to handle crises with positivity and to maintain harmony. During the Edo period, the Samurai Shogunate had governed and feudal lords had held power, yet the Samurai government was sanctioned by the Emperor and the power of the feudal lords borrowed from the Emperor. The restoration of imperial rule in 1867 required that all power be transferred back to the Emperor in order to unify Japan. There are few, if any, other countries that could experience such a transfer of power so smoothly.

The most recent example was the 1945 defeat in the Pacific War. In Japan, World War II is known as the Pacific War because Japan was not involved in any European battles. In the American occupation following their defeat, Japan faced many changes and enforced renouncement of its ancient culture which you can learn more about in Chapter 8. Despite this, and despite the loss of 700,000 innocent civilians during the bombing campaigns, the postwar occupation was carried out surprisingly smoothly, without resistance or internal conflict. Plus, no-one could have anticipated the following economic recovery after such a difficult occupation.

Though these events were tough and brought negative aspects with them, Japanese people managed to keep harmony throughout and to remain positive. They were flexible enough to use the situations to create something new by allowing the foreign cultures and ideas to merge with existing Japanese culture and values. Herein lies the strength of the Japanese and the reason they have survived as a country for more than

2,000 years.

## Folk remedies and alternative healing therapies

Few people in Japan realize that in the late Meiji to early Showa eras, Japan was quite advanced in terms of spirituality (Hirotsugu Imura *New: Feast of Miraculous-Method Practitioners* "新・霊術家の宴" ISBN 488302248X). This is not surprising because Shinto is rich in spirituality, both in essence and thought, and fostered a variety of healing techniques in its long history (Motohisa Yamakage *The Essence of Shinto* ISBN 1568364377 - English edition). Various folk remedies and alternative therapies were also regularly used in this prewar period along with acupuncture and many therapists known as *Reijutsu-ka* (霊術家, professionals who can use mysterious techniques).

These days, Japanese enjoy a nationwide medical insurance system that started in 1958. Almost everyone has their own doctor and can receive examinations and treatments under this insurance covering 70-80% of the cost. However, during the Meiji period, when the government was keen to introduce the Western medical system (based on the German system at the time), people had to pay 100% of the expensive medical costs. As a result of this, alternative therapies played an important role during these eras and people depended largely on them alongside folk remedies and sometimes even incantations and prayers. Shinto shrines, Buddhist temples and *Shugendo* (修験道, Japanese mountain asceticism and shamanism incorporating Shinto and Buddhist concepts) often provided health care services too, though these most likely had a wide range of effectiveness. In

1882 (Meiji 15) the government banned, *treatment solely using incantations and prayers without medical treatment or prescribed medicine*. The fact that the government saw fit to ban them means such treatments were common at the time. The ban can't have been wholly successful either because people were still using incantations and prayers just after the end of the Pacific War.

## Official health care providers

There were a wide range of recognized health care providers in the Meiji period. The first government survey of them in 1873 (Meiji 6) showed there being 28,262 providers - about 81 providers per 100,000 people (the total population of Japan at that time was 35,000,000) However, *only 20% of the providers had Western medical training*. Most of them were herbal doctors of Chinese medicine. Some of the providers had not had comprehensive training, they had started their medical care by reading introductory medical literature and a few couldn't even write (Yasuhiko Fukuda *National Qualification of Medical Doctors*, Hiroshima-city report 2003).

Other medical statistics of a prefectural area in Japan show some interesting changes across the Meiji and Taisho periods. Statistics in Saga prefecture in 1884 (Meiji 17) indicate there were 728 Western medical doctors at the time, 260 traditional Japanese midwives, 185 acupuncturists and 101 Chinese herbal pharmacists. Though there is an increase in the percentage of Western medical doctors by this time, a significant percentage of these professional medical providers still weren't using Western medicine. 30 years on, during the Taisho era (1912-1926) the number of traditional Japanese midwives had increased to more than 500 and the number of acupuncturists had increased to more than 700 while the number of Western doctors stayed about the same. This is fascinating. So many non-Western health care providers were being used although there must have been ambiguity around what was officially a medical treatment and what was an alternative therapy. As I mentioned above, the lack of insurance and high costs of Western treatment must have played a large part in this.

## The surge of Reijutsu-ka

A broad range of alternative therapies came about during these prewar eras. Though they were new, their origins were based in Shugendo, Esoteric Buddhism and old Shinto techniques. Practitioners of these therapies were known as Reijutsu-ka where *Rei* (霊) means mysterious, *jutsu* (術) means technique, and *ka* (家) means professional. Literature A describes these in more detail. They most likely developed as a reaction to the government's attempts to westernize Japanese culture. People were not going to take on the Western medical system easily, plus they needed affordable daily health care.

Famous Reijutsu-ka awakened many followers who succeeded them. There were a surprising number of books and magazines about Reijutsu, some of which have been reprinted today. Interestingly, these publications present spiritual concepts and a worldview very similar to those of modern Western spiritualism. Japanese people were already absorbed in such spiritual concepts long before Western spirituality was imported after the

25

war. The use of such alternative therapies by the Japanese population, and the spiritual concepts that came with them was highly progressive compared to other countries of the time.

## The emergence of new religions

The *Order to separate Shinto and Buddhism* in 1868 was the beginning of the *National Shinto* created by the Meiji government. National Shinto placed the Emperor at the centre to be worshipped and overruled the former independency of Shinto shrines and groups. The free spiritual nature of Shinto was suppressed and rituals standardized. The Emperor was now a living God under which all Japan could be controlled and mobilized for the coming war. This was not the Emperor's decision but one taken by the government.

As a consequence of this suppression of traditional Japanese culture and religious control by the Meiji government, many new religions emerged. Some people tried to encourage a move back to the old Shinto. People such as *Chika-atsu Honda* (本田親徳) and *Honji Kawatsura* (川面凡児) researched the original Shinto and wrote books on it. Others began new religions based on the old Shinto spirituality. Examples of this are *Tenri-kyo* (天理教), *Kurozumi-kyo* (黒住教), *Konkou-kyo* (金光教) and *Ohmoto-kyo* (大本教). The latter was one of the largest religious groups and was cracked down on by the government, later splitting to become *Sekai-Kyusei-kyo* (世界救世教) and *Seityou-no-ie* (生長の家) in order to survive (Hiromi Shimada *Ten new religions in Japan* "日本の10大新宗教" ISBN 4344980603).

These new religions also provided hand healing based on techniques inherited from old Shinto, Shugendo and *Mikkyo* (密教, Tantric Buddhism). They used both hands-on and non-touch therapies.

## Reiki

Mikao Usui started Reiki in the midst of all these political, health and social changes. It was the Taisho era when traditional medical therapies were increasing in response to the government attempt to normalize Western medical doctors. However, it's important to remember that Reiki had no direct connections with any of the religious healing techniques springing up at the time.

# Chapter 2 Reiki and The Beginning of Reiki as a Therapy

Hands-on therapies and healing have been commonly used across the world since ancient times. In this sense, they are not unusual or special in the way people often think of them today. As far back as the sixth century in Japan, *Onmyoji* (陰陽師), a professional practitioner of esoteric cosmology, used hands-on therapy as a medical treatment. Old Shinto seems to have used hands-on therapies too. In fact, the Japanese language itself indicates that such therapy has been used since ancient times - the Japanese word for 'treatment' is *Teate* (手当て), which when directly translated means 'hands-on'. *Te* (手) means 'hand' and *ate* (当て) means 'apply' or 'put-on' so the very concept of treatment must have begun with hands-on therapy in Japan.

## Is Reiki just another hands-on therapy?

There are several characteristics that clearly differentiate Reiki from all other hands-on therapies, both older therapies and those used by the Reijutsu-ka (professionals using mysterious techniques) that sprung up in the 1920s and 1930s. Practitioners of hands-on therapies were those special few who were extensively trained or even enlightened. Many people are familiar with various methods used by these Reijutsu-ka such as qigong, yell therapy, hypnotherapy, hand healing and religious faith-healing. However, Reiki therapy, started by Mikao Usui (臼井甕男1865-1926, hereafter Usui) had nothing to do with these practices and was not related to any religion. It was born entirely independently and discovered unintentionally. Usui would have known about the Reijutsu-ka and religious healings of his day. His varied work as a public official, a businessman, a journalist and secretary to a politician would have meant he was familiar with current news and affairs and both Reijutsu-ka and new religions often appeared in the newspapers of the day. Mikao Usui discovered and established Reiki independently of all these. He found Reiki quite by chance when he injured his foot climbing down the mountain after fasting on *Mt.Kurama* (鞍馬山) in northern Kyoto in 1922. If he had been searching for a healing method it would have been impossible for him to discover Reiki. I know this is a bold statement to make, but hopefully the information in this and the following chapter will help you to understand why this is true.

## Unique characteristics of Reiki

Reiki is an innate ability that anyone can use, everyone has the chance to be a Reiki therapist for their parents, children and friends! To discover this was truly revolutionary and represented a significant divergence from previous therapies. The Reijutsu-ka hand healings made use of *energy intentionally created by practitioners* - very similar to qigong methods. I have read a variety of literature from that time and not one author understood the difference between energy used in qigong and Reiki energy. Even for Japanese people at that time it was not easy to recognize that *Reiki flows through every human body naturally, without them needing to do anything*. This energy can be effectively used to heal diseases.

Another important characteristic of Reiki is that it is not connected to religion. Many hands-on therapies were religious and needed the practitioner to believe in God or dogma of some kind. However, Reiki was established without any religious requirement, and because there is no need to believe in anything to practice Reiki, it can be used freely by everyone.

The Reijutsu-ka, who had a strong intention to heal or change someone, and the religious people, who pre-required certain beliefs, could not possibly have perceived Reiki as it is, because it flows out unconsciously without any intention or beliefs.

To allow people to begin using Reiki easily and quickly, Usui sensei created *Reiju* (霊授), known in Western Reiki as an 'attunement'. This technique was pioneering compared with other therapies as they required lengthy training before anyone could practice.

---

In summary:

- Everyone can use Reiki

- One does not need to be a saint

- One does not have to believe in anything

- One does not use one's own energy

- A one day seminar is enough to start Reiki

- Reiki is so easy, even children can use it

---

Though there have been many hands-on therapies established across a variety of eras and a wide range of countries, Reiki is the first therapy to possess all these characteristics. Usui had to be independent of all the

Reijutsu-ka and religions to discover Reiki and was wise enough to allow Reiki to be what it is and not attempt to make it fit with what he already knew.

The full name for Reiki is *Shin-shin Kaizen Usui Reiki Ryou-ho* (心身改善 白井靈氣療法) where *Shin-shin* (心身) means 'mind & body', *Kaizen* (改善) means 'to improve', *Reiki* (靈氣) means 'invisible energy with miraculous power', and *Ryou-ho* (療法) means 'therapy'.

**Common misunderstandings about Reiki**

**1. Usui wanted to heal like Jesus**

Some Western Reiki authors have stated that Usui had been searching for a healing method that replicated the healing Jesus or Buddha performed. There is no evidence that supports this story. The fact that Usui engaged in the kind of work he did and that he repeatedly changed his work before finally confining himself to a zen temple for three years indicates he was heading in a different direction than finding a healing therapy method. The story is just a fable created by Hawayo Takata in order to have a greater impact on her Western students when she taught them (I write more about Hawayo Takata in Chapter 9).

In addition, as I mentioned previously, it is highly unlikely that anyone searching for a healing method would come across Reiki because the act of searching and trying is contrary to the state one needs to be in to allow Reiki to flow.

## 2. A book about Reiki was published in 1914

An internet rumor exists that a Japanese man called *Mataji Kawakami* (川上又次) published a book titled *Reiki Therapy and its Effects* in 1914, eight years before Usui discovered Reiki. However, no one has ever seen or read this book, it has yet to be found if it does actually exist, which I doubt. If it is ever found, I would be interested to see if and how it related to Usui's Reiki.

## 3. Reiki originated in Tibet

Other Western Reiki authors have claimed that Reiki originated in Tibet. This is untrue and none of these authors have found any evidence to support their claims. This misunderstanding probably comes from the fact that one of the Reiki symbols Usui designed comes from *Bonji* (梵字), which is a type of Sanskrit lettering that originated in Northern India and was imported into Japan in the seventh century. These days in India Bonji has been replaced by a more modern type of writing while in Japanese Buddhism it is still used. Aside from Usui taking the inspiration for one symbol from Sanskrit there is no direct or indirect connection between Sanskrit and Reiki.

## 4. Reiki energy is related to Mt. Kurama

Mt. Kurama (鞍馬, where *Kura* 鞍 means saddle and *ma* 馬 means house) seems to occupy a privileged place among many Reiki practitioners. This is because they blindly relate Reiki to Mt. Kurama without fully understanding what Reiki really is. Despite Usui being on the mountain when he discovered the existence of Reiki energy, *Mt. Kurama has no special relationship with Reiki itself or with symbols used in Reiki techniques.*

To ordinary Japanese, Mt. Kurama and its temple are simply famous for the legend of *Ushiwaka-maru* (牛若丸) a young samurai who was taught martial arts by the long-nosed goblin of Mt. Kurama. The story is written in famous literature of the Heian-era (8th - 12th century) such as *The Tale of Genji* and *The Pillow Book of Sei-Shonagon.*

The temple on Mt Kurama was initiated in 770 by *Kantei* (鑑禎), younger brother of *Kanjin* (鑑真), who worshipped *Bishamon-ten* (毘沙門天 The God of Treasure). Later, in 796, *Fujiwara-no-Isendo* (藤原伊勢人), who worshipped *Senju-kan-non* (千手観音 The thousand-armed God of Mercy, said to be the northern guard of Kyoto at the time) further established the basic functionality of the temple.

Kurama temple first belonged to the Tendai Buddhist sect, then it changed to the Shingon Buddhist sect and later returned to the Tendai sect. After that, during the postwar allied occupation, GHQ (the US occupation headquarters), began promoting the reorganization of religious groups. In 1947, Kurama temple established itself as having its own religion called *Kurama Koukyo* (鞍馬弘教). The temple detached from the Tendai sect and became the sole place of worship for Kurama Koukyo. At this time the God, *Goho-Maoson* (護法魔王尊, Sanat Kumara) was added to the temple and it was decided that the philosophy of Kurama temple would be to worship *Sonten* (尊天), a Trinity of three gods. The present Kurama temple still worships this Trinity as light, love and power - Bishamonten and Senju Kannon, who were connected to the temple in the eighth century and Maoson, who became connected to Kurama during the occupation after the Pacific War.

The doctrine of Kurama Koukyo is very different from that of Buddhism. It states, *"As our doctrine, we are to establish a Trinity, Sonten, which is the Great Spirit of the Universe, Dai-Koumyo (大光明, great enlightenment), and the Great Acting Embodiment. In other words, Sonten is the cosmic life and energy that creates all existence in this world. It is something appearing as energy that transcends both Buddhist and Shinto Gods."*

Someone in Western Reiki, attracted to the philosophy of Kurama Koukyo, mistakenly associated each Reiki symbol with the three Gods of this Trinity. In their enthusiasm, they introduced the fourth symbol as Sonten. However, as you can see, these associations have nothing to do with the original Reiki that Usui was practicing. Sonten, in the context of Mt Kurama, did not even come into existence until long after Usui's death in 1926.

The doctrine of Kurama Koukyo sounds more like new age thought than religion. *Shin-gaku Kou-un* (信楽香雲), the head of Kurama temple and founder of Kurama Koukyo, studied 19th century Western theosophy before he established Kurama Koukyo which is probably one of the reasons why the religion goes well with new age thought and Western Reiki. I have observed that Western people generally favor a well-defined single system over seemingly unrelated individual components - in other words, they prefer to have a single God and the idea that the three Gods form one as a Trinity would therefore be appealing.

Mt. Kurama, its temple, Gods and shrine are all quite fascinating. However, Reiki itself has no intrinsic relationship with religion or the Gods of Kurama. There is absolutely no need to believe in Kurama Koukyo, Reiki exists independently of our thoughts or beliefs. I can't emphasize enough that Mt Kurama has nothing to do with Reiki energy, it was Western Reiki practitioners who introduced the misguided relationship between Reiki energy and Mt Kurama.

## 5. Japanese culture - and therefore Reiki - is based on Buddhism

Non-Japanese often associate Japanese culture with Buddhism, probably because there is so much literature on Buddhism. They analyze Japan only by looking into the relationship between the two. Such an approach is not entirely mistaken, for Buddhism is firmly embedded in our culture now, however, when trying to understand Reiki, it's a limitation and many foreigners fail to grasp what Reiki truly is as a result.

Buddhism sits on a fundamental idea that life is pain and suffering. This contrasts strongly with Reiki which sees humans as capable of an inherently good and healthy existence. Rather than having roots in Buddhism, Reiki has more affinity with the original Japanese culture. Shinto is an example of this and Reiki is often consistent with the ideology and world view of traditional Shinto. The challenge comes with the fact that Shinto can be difficult to understand even for many Japanese. There is no dogma associated with Shinto, no manuscripts on it and very little written about it. It cannot be understood in terms of Western religion and mindset. If there is little available on traditional Shinto in Japanese, there is even less available to English speakers. I have not come across any foreign authors who have studied Reiki in terms of Shinto or old Japanese culture. I am going to look into Reiki and old Japanese culture in detail in a later chapter which I hope is helpful to you.

## 6. Reiki means 'Universal Life Force'

The word *Reiki* (靈氣) can be found in the common Japanese dictionary with an example such as *Reiki, the sacred energy, filling the deep forest. Rei* (靈) means mysterious, miraculous or sacred. (The kanji character, 靈 sometimes means spirit too). *Ki* (氣) means invisible energy. Therefore Reiki means *invisible energy with mysterious power.* The word 靈氣 (Reiki) is not necessarily always related to living things so translating it as *universal life force*, while not wrong per se, is not accurate as an explanation of the word. You will see Reiki written in kanji in two ways. 靈氣 is a traditional way of writing Reiki, while 靈気 is a modern version -- which one you use is just a matter of preference.

The word, Reiki, then, does not necessarily mean a hands-on therapy, so we often use the words *Reiki Ryoho* because *Ryoho* means *therapy.*

## Mikao Usui

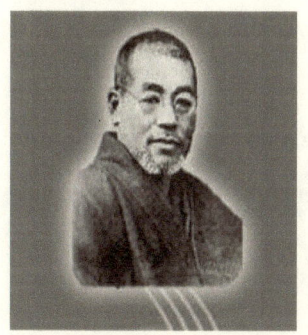

Mikao Usui was born in 1865 and died in 1926. He is known for discovering Reiki in 1922 by chance after fasting on Mt Kurama for a period of time. Little is known about Usui's life before the incident. His family roots stretch back to samurai warriors, the *Chiba* family, who were very active in the Heian to Kamakura period (8th - 14th century). Today one of the Japanese prefectures is called Chiba prefecture after this samurai clan.

Usui changed his occupation many times and was a public official, businessman, journalist, and secretary to a politician among other things. He sometimes visited abroad but left no written information about himself or any biography. He seemed to dislike talking about himself or being seen in public. There are only five photographs of him available today. One is in this book, one was taken with twenty *shihans* (teachers) just two months before his death, one is a portrait photo in a garden, and the last two are photographs with members of the *Usui Reiki Ryoho Gakkai* (臼井療法学会, hereafter known as *Gakkai*). Gakkai means society.

A few significant dates in his life are:

- March 1922: Found Reiki after fasting on Mt. Kurama.
- April 1922: Established Gakkai in *Harajuku, Tokyo* and started Reiki therapy and teaching.

- February 1924: Moved to *Nakano, Tokyo*.
- March 9th 1926: Died in *Fukuyama, Hiroshima* at the age of 62.

As you can see, he started Reiki therapy and teaching only one month after finding Reiki on Mt. Kurama. His enlightenment may well have enabled such a quick move.

Two years after Usui's death, his pupils erected a large stone monument alongside his tombstone with an inscription about how Usui lived. The epitaph on the stone was written in old-style formal Japanese and is therefore very difficult for present Japanese people to understand. Though a few experts have translated it into modern Japanese, my father, who also happens to be an expert on 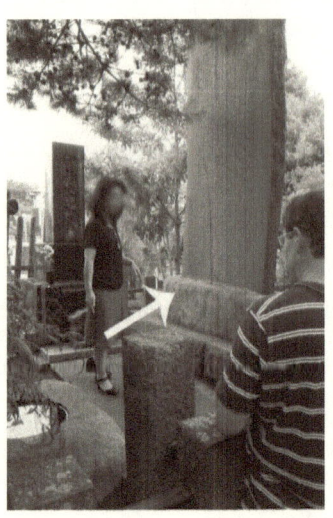 such things, kindly gave me an independent translation. I have translated his version into English below.

(The Japanese language is written vertically from top to bottom with columns read from right to left.)

# 霊法肇祖臼井先生功徳之碑

白井先生功徳碑

夫レ修養練磨ノ実ヲ積ミテ中ニ得ル所アルヲ之ヲ徳ト謂ヒ開導拯済ノ道ヲ弘メテ外ニ施ス所アルヲ之ヲ功ト謂フ功高ク徳大ニシテ始メテ一大宗師タルコトヲ得ベシ古来ノ賢哲俊徳ノ士学統ヲ樹テ宗旨ヲ創メシ者ハ皆然ラサルハナシ臼井先生ノ如キモ亦其ノ人ナルカ先生新ニ宇宙ノ霊気ニ本ヅキ心身ヲ善クスル法ヲ肇ム四方伝ヘ聞キ教ヲ乞ヒ療ヲ願フ者蝟然トシテ之ニ帰ス嗚呼亦盛ンナルカナ先生通称甕男号ハ暁帆岐阜県山県郡谷合村ノ人其ノ先ハ千葉常胤ニ出ツ父諱ハ胤氏通称宇左衛門俗ハ河合氏先生慶応元年八月十五日ヲ以テ生レ幼ヨリ苦学力行衆ニ超ユ長スルニ及ビ欧米ニ航シ支那ニ游ブ既ニシテ世ニ立ツ志ト違ヒ轗軻不遇歴窮約ニ処シ然レトモ竟ニ屈撓セス嘗テ鞍馬山ニ登リ食ヲ断チテ苦学辛練スルコト二十有一日ニ候チテ一大霊気ヲ頭上ニ感シ忽然トシテ霊気療法ヲ得タリ是ヨリ之ヲ身ニ試ミ試ニ家人ニ験スルニ効効立チトコロニ見ハル先生以為ヘラク独リ其ノ家人ニ善クスルヨリ広ク世人ニ授ケテ其ニ及ボサント乃チ慶ニ頗ルニ若カスト大正十一年四月居ヲ東京青山原宿ニ定メ学会ヲ設ケ霊気療法ヲ行フ遠近来リ乞フ者廬戸外ニ満ツ十二年九月大震火災起リ創傷病苦至ル処ニ呻吟ス先生深ク之ヲ痛ミ日ニ出テテ市ヲ巡リ救療スルコト幾何ナルヲ知ルヘカラス其ノ急ニ赴キ患ヲ済フコト大率此ノ如シ後道場ヲ狭隘ナリトシ十四年二月市外中野ニ築キ声誉弥々著ハレ地方ヨリ招聘スル者少カラス先生其ノ需ニ応シテ呉ニ又広島ニ向ヒ佐賀ニ入リ尋テ福山ニ抵ル偶疾病ニ罹リ遂ニ其ノ地ニ歿ス時ニ大正十五年三月九日ナリ享年六十二配鈴木氏名ハ貞子一男二女ヲ生ム男ハ不二ヲ曰ヒ家ヲ嗣グ先生人トナリ温厚恭謙ヲ以テ本トシ辺幅ヲ飾ラス躯幹肥大豊ニシテ笑ヲ含ミ其ノ事ニ当ルヤ剛毅ニシテ善ク忍ヒ用意尤モ深キ人トナリ才芸多ク書ヲ好ミ史伝ニ渉リ医道ノ書ニ及ヒ仏耶ノ経典ニ出入シ心理ノ学神仙ノ方禁呪占筮相人ノ術ニ至ルマテ通セサルナシ蓋シ先生ノ好ム所ノ学芸経歴八修養練磨ノ資料トナリ修養練磨八霊法開創ノ管鍵トナリシコト論ヲ俟タサルナリ先生曰ク霊法八天賦ノ霊能ニ因リテ心正シク身健カニ人生ノ福祉ヲ享ケシムルニ在リ故ニ其ノ人ヲ教フルヤ先ツ明治天皇ノ遺詠ヲ奉体シ朝夕五戒ヲ唱ヘテ心ニ念シ念シ二日ニ三日今日怒ルナカレ心配スルナカレ感謝シテ業ヲ励メ人ニ親切ナレト是レ実ニ修養ノ一大訓ニシテ古聖賢ノ警戒スルモノ其ノ揆ヲ一ニセリ先生之ヲ以テ招福ノ秘法ヲ日ク人ニ親切ナレ其ノ本領ノ在ル所知ルヘシ又其ノ教フルヤ簡易ニシテ愛フル勿ク一日ニシテ克ク五官ノ病ヲ除去シ先生曰ク靈能力ヲ以テ人心ヲ收攬シ以テ靈能ニ導クガ故ニ其ノ人ヲ教フルヤ先ツ明治天皇ノ遺詠ヲ奉体シ朝夕念誦ニ醇健ノ心ヲ養ヒ平正ノ行ニ復セシムルニ在リ是レ靈法ノ何人モ企及シ易キ所以ナリ挽近世遠ク古ニ遡リ既往ヲ稽シ将来ヲ念フノ思想ノ変動漸クカラス擧ゲテ此ノ靈法ヲ普及シ以テ人心ノ改善ヲ図ラント欲スル者アリ道場ニ会シテ遺薬ヲ継キ地方ニ在ルモ亦各其ノ法ヲ伝フ先生近クト雖モ靈法ハ永ク世ニ宣播スヘシ嗚呼先生ノ中ニ得テ外ニ施ス者豈ニ亦大ナラスヤ頃者門下ノ諸士相議シ石ヲ豎テ其ノ功徳ヲ頌シテ以テ不朽ニ図ラント文ヲ予ニ属シ予深ク先生ノ偉蹟ニ服シ諸士ノ篤ヲ嘉シ敢テ辞セスシテ其ノ梗概ヲ叙シ後人ヲシテ観感瞻仰スル能ハサラシメンコトヲ庶幾フ

昭和二年二月

従三位勲三等文学博士　岡田正之撰
海軍少将従四位勲三等功四級　牛田従三郎書

---

The Founder of A Miraculous Therapy

Monument to The Accomplishment and Virtue of Master Usui.

*Virtue* is to achieve inner fulfillment through cultivating one's life and training one's mind. *Accomplishment* is to benefit society by paving the way, leading others to liberation.

One can be a great leader in a given field only if one's virtue is high and accomplishment great. All great and wise persons are able to build new creations upon the foundation of authentic knowledge that came before them because of their virtue and accomplishment. Master Usui was one of these.

He developed a new method to heal mind and body based on the Reiki that fills the Universe. The atmosphere around him was vibrant because so many people were drawn to the master to learn the method and to receive treatment.

Mikao (臼井甕男) is his given first name and Gyohan (暁帆) his pen name. He was born in Taniai village, Yamagata City, Gifu prefecture and came from the lineage of Tsunetane Chiba (千葉常胤 1118 - 1201) [Author's note: Chiba was a samurai who supported Yoritomo Minamoto, the Shogun in 12th century].

His father was known as Uzaemon (宇左衛門) but his real name was Uzitane (胤氏), while his mother's family name was Kawai (河合).

Master Usui was born on August 15th 1865. Because he faced challenges during his childhood and worked diligently through school, his level of study became more advanced than that of his friends.

As an adult he visited Europe and the United States and studied in China. In society, his experience was different from his vision. His wish was unfulfilled and he was undervalued, occasionally reduced to poverty. In the face of such challenges, he did not give up and continued to discipline himself.

On one occasion, he climbed Mt Kurama and started fasting and meditating for 21 days.

One day he felt great Reiki energy on his head. Through this awakening and enlightening experience, he came to understand Reiki therapy. He explored its effectiveness by experimenting on himself and his family, then decided it was best to share the therapy widely, with all people not just his family.

In April 1922 (Taisho 11), he settled in Harajuku, Aoyama, Tokyo. He founded a society, taught Reiki therapy and gave treatments. So many people came to him from near and far that the entrance overflowed with visitors' shoes. [Author's note: In Japan, people take off their shoes at the entrance of a house.]

In September 1923 (Taisho 12), the *Great Kanto Earthquake* struck. In the disaster area [Author's note: The earthquake hit Tokyo] there were injured, groaning and suffering people everywhere. This made Master Usui's heart ache terribly and from that morning he travelled the area giving treatments and saving countless people. This was how he contributed during such a sudden disaster.

His school needed to expand after this, and he acquired land in Nakano, suburban Tokyo, chosen as a result of his divining skills. He built a new school there in February 1925 (Taisho 14).

As his reputation grew, he was often invited to provinces such as Kure, Hiroshima and Saga. On March 9th, 1926 (Taisho 15), during a visit to Fukuyama, he became unexpectedly ill and died at the lodgings he was staying in. He was 62.

His wife's name was Sadako (貞子); her maiden name was Suzuki (鈴木). They had a son and two daughters. The son, Fuji (不二) was successor of the Usui line.

Master Usui was a gentle, humble and unpretentious man. He was stocky and well-built. He always dealt with people with a smile, yet had deep concern when there was a problem and managed it using his strength and patience. He liked to read books about history, medical science, psychology, biographies, Buddhist sutras and the Christian Bible. In addition he was well-versed in the hermit technique of Taoism and and in divination. His wide range of knowledge and vast learning were the key to developing this *Reiho* (霊法) [Author's note: The memorial stone uses the word *Reiho*, meaning *miraculous method* to talk about Reiki therapy.]

The essence of *Reiho* is used not only to cure diseases but also to become healthy in body and mind, and to use the heaven-sent, miraculous ability within us to enjoy the happiness of life. The master therefore told his pupils to carry out the teachings of the Meiji Emperor and to keep *Gokai* [the five principles] in their heart and mind by chanting it morning and evening.

The first principle is not to become angry [today]
The second is not to worry [today]
The third is to be grateful [today]
The fourth is to devote yourself to what you need to do [today]
The fifth is to be kind to people [today]

*Gokai* is truly a great teaching to cultivate one's life, in accord with the counsel of past wise sages. The master regarded *Gokai* as a secret method to invite happiness and mysterious medicine to cure diseases. This demonstrates his true ability.

When he taught *Gokai*, he used familiar examples and avoided complicated expressions, explaining it in simple terms. In this way, he led people to truth. Chanting *Gokai* morning and evening in *seiza* [Author's note: sitting on one's heels] and *gassho* [Author's note: putting ones' palms together] brings one to engage in daily life with a calm mind and a pure heart. In this way, everyone can easily practice *Reiho*.

The purpose of this Reiho is not solely to cure diseases or serious illnesses. In today's rapidly changing society, it can be challenging to maintain a peaceful heart and mind. The spread of this Reiho would help enormously to stabilize society and calm people.

Master Usui has more than 2,000 students and his leading disciples continue to gather in the Tokyo school and teach in areas all around Japan. Even after his death, Reiho will continue and the seeds sown will be widespread.

How wonderful that Master Usui acquired the truth of this Reiho within himself and chose to share it with others.

To commemorate and immortalize the accomplishment and virtue of Master Usui, some of his students decided to build this memorial at the graveyard of Saihouji Temple in Toyotama district, suburban Tokyo. I have been asked to write this epitaph. I appreciate the strong relationship he had with his students and I myself benefit from the great legacy left by Master Usui, so I happily accepted their request and here outline the Master's life and his exceptional work.

I hope that coming generations read this monument and do not forget what is written here.

February 1927 (Showa 2)
Composed by

Doctor of Literature, *Masayuki Okada* (岡田正之)

(Junior third rank of honor, awarded the third order)

Calligraphed by

Rear Admiral, *Jyuzaburo Ushida* (牛田従三郎)

(Junior fourth rank of honor, awarded the third order, awarded the fourth military order)

[Author's note: The official rank of honor was given by the Imperial court while the the third and fourth orders were medals presented by the government in the presence of the Emperor].

The epitaph was created by Masayuki Okada (1864 -1927), a scholar of Chinese writing who was born in Toyama. He first became a professor at Army Cadet School, then a professor at Gakushuin University and in 1924 a professor at the University of Tokyo. The Gakkai consisted of many people of such a high social status. He died in the same year this memorial stone was erected.

Usui's tombstone is visited by a huge number of foreign Reiki practitioners these days; the wish of his pupils really did come true.

### Reiki practitioners of the time - Numbers

Let me estimate the minimum number of Reiki practitioners at that time. A few member lists for Usui's Gakkai were discovered by someone browsing through a used book store quite by chance. They indicate that in 1926 the number of members was about 2,000, in 1928 it was 5,000 and by 1930 had reached 7,000. Given the speed at which the numbers were increasing, I would say there were probably more than 10,000 Gakkai members by the time Japan entered the war. There were independent practitioners in addition to the Gakkai members, some of whom had withdrawn from the Gakkai. These included *Chujiro Hayashi* (林忠治郎), *Kaiji Tomita* (冨田魁二) and *Toshihiro Eguchi* (江口俊博).

Usui strictly forbade open publicity and advertisements in the Gakkai allowing it to spread only by word of mouth. Meanwhile, the independent Tomita and Eguchi made use of advertisements and gave open seminars in an effort to spread Reiki. Hayashi regularly gave seminars in Tokyo, Osaka and sometimes in local districts too, taking care of many students. These independent teachers probably created a similar number of Reiki practitioners to that of the Gakkai which would make the number of Reiki practitioners in Japan before the war somewhere around 50,000.

If we include numbers of other, non-Reiki, hands-on practitioners (including Reijutsu-ka and those in religions) there may have been in order of 100,000 hands-on practitioners. This number is significant because the present number of Japanese and Western Reiki practitioners in Japan is often quoted as being just over 50,000. Considering the population of Japan is currently twice what it was before the war, there can be no doubt that hands-on therapies were more popular before than after the war. Some of my Reiki students have grandparents who were practicing hands-on therapies before the war. I'll talk more about this in a later Chapter.

## Reiki practitioners of the time - Support from Naval officers

A number of naval officers played important roles in the Gakkai. At least five of the 20 shihans (teachers) Usui taught were high-ranking naval officers (Toshitaka Mochizuki *Reiki: iyashino-te* ASIN B01KWJ9XI8). After Usui's death, Juzaburo Ushida (1865-1935), a rear admiral and the man to calligraph Usui's memorial stone, became the second president. Another rear admiral followed him as president, *Kanichi Taketomi* (武富咸一 1878-1960) and while the fourth was not a naval man, after the war, former vice admiral *Houichi Wanami* (和波豊一1883-1975) became the fifth president.

A rear admiral is often the highest officer commanding a major battle ship, and a vice admiral sometimes serves as a governmental committee member. Chujiro Hayashi, who was a trustee of the Gakkai, was a naval colonel. Hayashi, as I will explain later, created opportunities for Reiki to spread abroad and for Jikiden Reiki to be accessible to people today.

The Gakkai had a branch at every major naval port such as Hiroshima, Kure, Sasebo and Ohminato. The Japanese Navy was relatively liberal but no-one is certain as to why Reiki was so popular among the officers. It is not outlandish to surmise that they had strategic reasons for its use. I had the chance to talk with a retired US Naval officer who trained the Japanese Navy in the

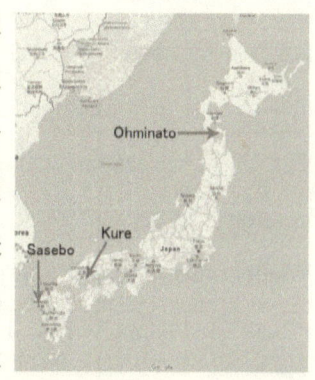

Kure Naval port in October, 1945. Most of ships are Navy ships.

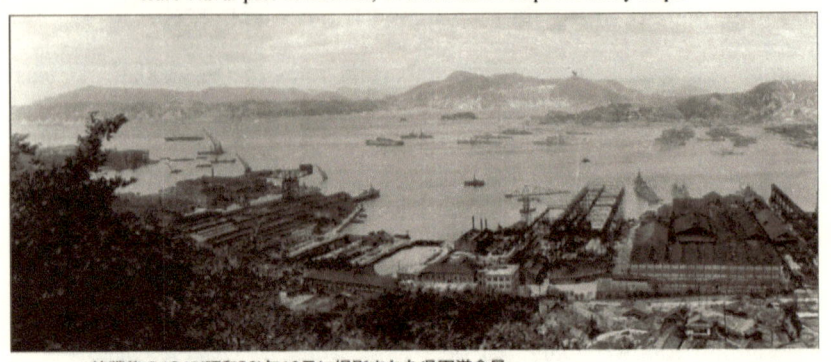

終戦後の1945(昭和20)年10月に撮影された呉軍港全景。
写真裏には「停泊するのは帝国船艇。左端は日本航空母艦鳳翔。
右端は爆撃で炎上した呉市。中央手前は呉海軍工廠」と記載されている（2枚のつなぎ写真）

1930s (I was surprised that the US and Japan had such close relationship before parting ways in the run up to the war). He explained that the Japanese Navy at that time was advanced both in terms of technology and strategy. It would therefore not be surprising if they had made the decision to use Reiki to treat sick and injured crew. In an isolated environment such as a battleship, only a limited amount of medicine would be available once the ship had left port. Battleships tended to be at sea for extensive periods of time, so chances to replenish stocks would be few and far between and they would want to save as much medicine and medical supplies as possible for actual battles. If Reiki was used on such a ship, they would be able to save medical supplies and maintain the health of the crew on board. This is, however, conjecture; there is no recorded evidence of Reiki being used on a battleship.

Whether this is true or not, Reiki was definitely used by high-ranking naval officers and supported by the Japanese Navy, a large national organization.

## Reiki practitioners of the time - Reiki used for treating diseases

In contrast to some types of Western Reiki today, where it is rarely used to help medical conditions, Reiki during this time was used as a powerful treatment for diseases. Of course the practitioners also understood that Reiki would improve their spiritual awareness but the majority of the time, it was used to treat disease and cure the sick.

Hayashi had his Reiki clinic in Tokyo's Shinano-machi, Shinjuku, where he had eight treatment beds and 16 Reiki therapists. Two therapists took care of one person typically spending 30 to 60 minutes with each client. They provided Reiki sessions in the morning in the clinic and then in the afternoon they were dispatched to treat people in other places. This information comes from *Hawayo Takata* and is probably pretty accurate because she worked at Hayashi's clinic for a half year as an intern. [Fran Brown *Living Reiki: Takata's Teachings* ISBN: 0940795108]

I write a little about Hayashi in Chapter 5 but cannot divulge everything because Hayashi's story is part of the Jikiden Reiki curriculum. Interested readers however, should consult the following books:

- Tadao Yamaguchi *Light on the Origins of Reiki* ISBN 0914955659
- Frank Arjava Petter *The Hayashi Reiki Manual* ISBN 0914955756

## Reiki practitioners of the time - Houichi Wanami

(和波豊一 1883 - 1975)

Wanami graduated from the 32nd class of the Naval Academy at the same time as *Isoroku Yamamoto* (Yamamoto is famous in Japan as the admiral who commanded the attack on Pearl Harbour). Wanami was a vice admiral and captain of a battleship and two submarine supply ships. He became principal of the Submarine Academy and was a member of the committee for the Ministry of Health and Welfare before the war.

Wanami was an expert in submarine tactics. The Naval Submarine Academy, where the operation of submarines was taught, was located in Kure until 1942. He became a teacher there, vice-principal, then principal from 1922 to 1934. During active service he commanded *Tokitukaze* (destroyer), *Komabashi* (sub. tender) and *Jingei* (sub. tender) successively.

Although it is not clear exactly when Wanami joined the Gakkai, it was definitely before 1926 because he is in the picture taken that year with Usui and other shihan members. Despite being assigned to reserve duty in 1936, he was sent to Hainan Island during the war. The island, as big as Taiwan, which is located further south-west, was Japanese territory at the

time and strategically important in terms of a southern advance when war broke out. The submarine base and corps on the island played an important role during the war until things changed towards the end and the island was no longer considered to be on the front line, producing coal mines instead.

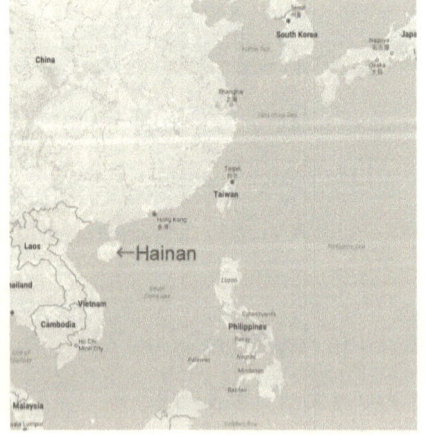

Although Wanami was already 53 years old when assigned to reserve duty, and 57 at the start of the war, he was so experienced as a captain and principal that he was sent to work at a crucially important base.

After the war, he served as fifth president of Usui's Gakkai, following *Yoshiharu Watanabe* (渡辺良治 ? - 1960) as the fourth. He led for the longest period of all the presidents, and during a particularly challenging time for Reiki. He ran the Gakkai together with Kimiko Koyama (小山君子) who became the succeeding president. During this period, in 1974, the important, *Reiki Therapy Brochure*, was published by the Gakkai.

In Chapter 8, I tell the story of how Wanami's family made use of Reiki after the war.

## Reiki practitioners of the time - Gizou Tomabechi
### (苫米地義三 1880 - 1959)

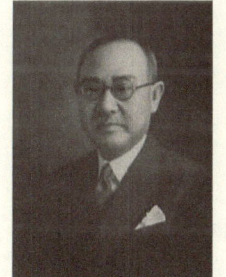

Tomabechi, a Dai-Shihan (senior teacher) of the Gakkai, was president of a fertilizer company before later becoming a politician. He became Minister of Transport in 1947-48, and both Secretary of State and Chief Cabinet Secretary of the following cabinet in 1948. In 1951, when Japan was released from occupation, he was the plenipotentiary for the opposition party during the San Francisco Peace Treaty (a plenipotentiary is a politician who can negotiate with foreign governments and sign treaties).

This picture shows the prime minister, Shigeru Yoshida, signing the treaty. Also in the frame, left to right are the politicians Tokugawa, Hoshijima, Tomabechi (indicated by the arrow) and Hayato Ikeda. [Photo from the Diplomatic Archive of the Ministry of Foreign Affairs, Japan].

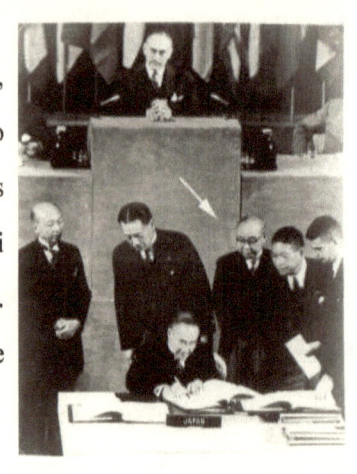

He published his biography in 1951 in which he writes about Reiki in a supplemental chapter. He speaks of Usui treating a woman patient in the excerpt below: (The picture shows Tomabechi treating a client.)

療を施したのであった。

もまだ呼びよせなかった宿屋住居であったので、治療所を設け、弟子も二三人おいて、無料治

かくて、世の人助けにもならばと折よく大日本人造肥料の関西部長として赴任早々で、家族

たりに旱た氏は、爾後この道の研究に精進し、ついに大師範の免許を師から受けたのである。

の夫は勿論、苦米地氏もしばし呆然として声も出なかった。この玄妙不可思議の霊法を目のあ

とすれば、これこそは正しく奇蹟だ。臼井氏はこれを見てただ笑っていたが、病人やその

あったが、病人は夫の肩に手をもたせかけながら歩き出した。

奇蹟ということが世にある

と、命じた。部屋は八畳で

「歩いて見なさい」

た。それを見て臼井氏は、

られた本人は「はい」と答えると同時にシャンと立上った。

と、言った。寝返りも出来ず一年も臥せていた病人にこういうことは無茶だと思ったが命ぜ

「起きて見なさい」

病人の腰を二三十分あまり治療した後、

が、一年位腰が立たぬということを聞き氏は、臼井氏に同道を願って治療に行った。臼井氏は

それはともかく、臼井式電気療法を研究し始めた頃、氏の会社の天海という会計係の妻君

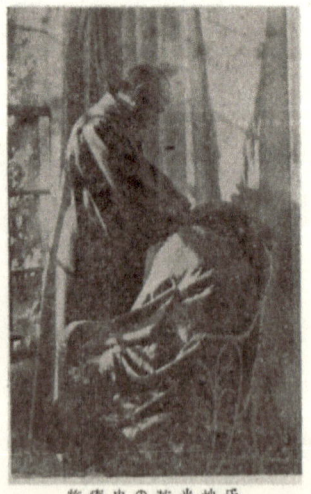

施療中の苫米地氏

It was when I started studying Usui Reiki Therapy. The wife of Mr. *Amami* (天海), an accountant in my company, was suffering greatly with a lower back problem and had been unable to stand up for a year. I asked Master Usui if he would give her treatment and so we went to see her. After treating her for 20 - 30 minutes, he said, "Try to stand up."

I thought it was absurd to say that to a sick person who had difficulty even turning over and had been laying in bed for a year. She, however, said, "Yes" as she stood up. She surprised herself by standing up! Watching her do so, Master Usui said, "Try to walk."

In a room the size of eight tatami mats, she started to walk with her hand on her husband's shoulder.

If there is something called a miracle in this world, that was surely it. Master Usui was just smiling as he watched, while the wife, her husband and I were totally speechless. Having seen this miraculous effectiveness with my own eyes, I devoted myself to Reiki therapy and was finally certified as Dai-Shihan by Master Usui.

It was easy for me to setup a clinic because it was just after I moved for my work as the chief of Kansai area and I had more time because my family weren't there. Thus, hoping to help people, I started giving voluntary treatments with a few pupils of mine.

If you are an experienced Reiki practitioner, you may be familiar with such 'miraculous effectiveness' after your treatments. What was amazing though, was that Usui did that just in 20 - 30 minutes.

# Chapter 3   Other Hands-on Therapies in Japan

Let's look at some of the other hands-on therapies in greater depth.

Firstly I'm going to explore two therapies originated by people who had previously learned Usui Reiki. Subsequently, I'll examine three of the Reijutsu (miraculous method) therapies that are unrelated to Reiki.

Of course there were many more hands-on therapies in existence, however, my intention is to give you an awareness of the kinds that were around in Japan and to see the similarities and differences between those and what Usui had discovered. *Doing this brings greater clarification of the fundamental characteristics of Usui Reiki.*

Many of the therapists have published their own books in Japanese, so I have studied those and, on occasion, personally explored their practical instructions to give you this information.

## Therapies originated by two former members of the Gakkai

1. *Kaiji Tomita* (富田魁二) - *Tomita-ryu Teate Ryoho* (富田流手当て 療法 - Tomita Hands-on Therapy)
2. Toshihiro Eguchi (江口俊博) - *Tenohira Ryoji* (手のひら療治 - Palm-on Therapy)

## 1. Kaiji Tomita - Tomita Hands-on Therapy

Tomita first learned Reiki in the Gakkai but became independent, founding

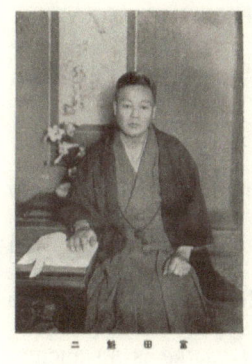

what he called, Tomita-ryu Teate Ryoho or Tomita Hands-on Therapy. His wonderful book, *Reiki to Ninjutsu* (Reiki and Compassion Technique) published in 1933 (Showa 8) is popular with many Japanese Jikiden Reiki practitioners. I recommend this book to anyone who would like to learn Reiki seriously. Sadly though, it is only available in Japanese at this time (ISBN 4894223368).

Tomita has given Reiki treatments to many people and emphasizes how important treatment practice is. He even provides statistics of the effectiveness of Reiki with various symptoms. Because the Reiki he practiced was very similar to what we practice as Japanese Reiki, his book is an excellent resource for Japanese Reiki practitioners.

Unfortunately, despite his wonderful work, he has no successors. One of his students, *Jiro Ashisuke* (足助次朗 1902-1986) who learned directly from Tomita in 1941 (Showa 16) published a book titled, *Teate Ryoho* (Hands-on Therapy, ISBN 4902271028) but the book shows that Ashisuke practiced very differently from his teacher. He seems to have developed his very own therapy.

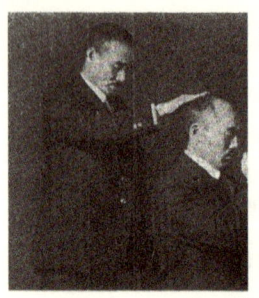

## 2. Toshihiro Eguchi - Tenohira Ryoji (Palm-on Therapy)

Eguchi (1873 - 1946) was a member of the Gakkai for two years before becoming independent and founding Tenohira Ryoji. He claimed it to be *Tanasue no Michi* (手末の道 The Way of Hands). *Tanasue* is an ancient way to say hand and by using it he was declaring that his method was developed in ancient times.

Others well-known for doing this therapy were:

· Koushi Mitsui (三井甲之 1883 - 1953)

  - Wrote the book *Tenohira Ryoho* (hands-on therapy ISBN 4902271001)

· Goro Miyazaki (宮崎五郎 ? - 1984)

  - An important successor of Eguchi's work

· Kou Kijima (喜島康, 1931 - )

  - The successor of Miyazaki's work

· Kazuo Mihashi (三橋一夫, 1928 - )

  - Wrote the book *Hands Cure illnesses* (ISBN 4813600476). Though there are several books on Eguchi's healing, Mihashi's book is the most concise and concrete. My description of Eguchi's therapy is based on this book.

Toshihiro Eguchi, born in 1873 (Meiji 6) in Kumamoto, the son of Army officer, suffered from injury, brain disease and pleurisy while he was young. After graduating from the Imperial University of Tokyo, he served as the high-school principal in Hiroshima, Nagano and Kofu. In 1926, at the age of 53, he became a member of the Gakkai, introduced by a woman named Tamura. He felt very uncomfortable about the expensive Gakkai admission fee of 50 yen which, based on the price of rice, would roughly correspond to 50,000 to 100,000 yen today (430 - 860 USD at the time of writing). Kaiji Tomita, who I mentioned above, had similar doubts about the admission fee.

Some Western books, such as *Reiki Sourcebook* by Bronwen Stiene and Frans Stiene (ISBN 1846941814) state Eguchi was a friend and classmate of Usui. However, there is no literature that proves their relationship and this information is probably false because if they had known each other Ms. Tamura would not have had to introduce him to the Gakkai.

Eguchi withdrew from the Gakkai in 1927. He thought it very unreasonable to make money on something given to everyone as a birthright. After becoming independent with his Tenohira Ryoji, many people came to his place to learn.

**Differences between Usui Reiki and Eguchi's therapy**
Looking at some fundamental characteristics of Eguchi's healing method, it is possible to see what Reiki is *not*. This contrast helps to further clarify what Reiki actually *is*.

Characteristics of Eguchi's method that **differ from Usui Reiki**:
*a) Therapist receives the client's energy*

While I agree with many aspects of Eguchi's thought, some I do not agree with. This is one of them. Eguchi believed that one would take on their client's karma if one accepted money in return for a treatment. He said, "You receive the client's energy because you become surrounded by the client's atmosphere." His student, Goro Miyazaki, took on the same idea. It is a flaw in his system to believe that a therapist will receive adverse effects from a client.

*b) Client needs to undergo preparation before a treatment*

The practitioner's hands are only applied after what is called *interchange* though the method for this is not indicated in the book. It is designed to soothe a client and help them relax. In Usui Reiki, applying the Reiki is what makes a client relax and soothes them so there is no need for preparation.

*c) Lack of method for improving spirituality*

Though Eguchi did recognize the importance of a practitioner's spirituality, there is no clearly proposed method to improve oneself other than composing poems, which seems a peculiar method to me. In Usui Reiki, enlightenment is an important theme from the outset. He came to establish Reiki in the process of achieving enlightenment and was clear that Reiki should be applied to mind and spirit. He named his therapy, Shin Shin Kaizen Usui Reiki Ryoho (Usui Reiki Therapy to Improve Mind and Body) where the first *shin* means *mind*. In addition, he introduced *Seiheki Chiryo* (性癖治療, treatment of mind habits) and Gokai (the five principles) where the former treats psychological problems and the latter is a guide into enlightenment.

*d) No indication that hands-on therapy has psychological effects*
The fact that Eguchi and Miyazaki's practitioners needed to prepare a client and calm them down before giving them treatment, rather than allowing the energy itself to do so indicates that they did not clearly recognize the psychological benefits of the energy on their clients. They do recognize that physical problems are often only temporarily cured unless psychological issues are also attended to, but they have no method to work directly on psychological problems either. For this reason, and those above, I do not think Eguchi's hands-on therapy is a solid, established system.

*e) Preconditions to a client receiving treatment*
In her book, *Tanagokoro* (Palm: ISBN 4773367903) the present successor, Kou Kijima writes, "I never offer my hands-on therapy to someone who does not practice what Master Miyazaki preached." In other words she would only treat those who were practicing. This is very strange to me, one cannot require such a precondition to a sick client.

*f) The practitioner cures the client - importance of hands*
In Eguchi's method, the practitioner's hands are regarded as extremely important. Hands appear to be the protagonists in the treatment and the cure, which keeps them stuck in the idea that the practitioner is central to curing the client. In Usui Reiki the practitioner's hands are not so important, they are simply one of the exits from which Reiki flows. What affects the client is not the hands, but the Reiki. The practitioner is not

curing the client, he or she cures him or herself using the Reiki energy - no matter where it comes out from. Usui clearly recognized the existence of the Reiki energy. This may be a subtle difference, but it is very important because it has a strong influence on how a practitioner will interact with a client.

*g) The energy flow is received through the hand*

Another thing that concerns me about Eguchi's therapy is the way they flow the energy. They receive it with the left hand and send it with the right. Miyazaki (his successor) also proposed a breathing practice called *Dondo no Kokyu* (呑吐の呼吸 - inhale and exhale breathing) where one receives the solar energy via the left hand and returns it to the universe through the right hand. In Usui Reiki, it is imperative that Reiki flows through one's **head** because of the positive effects that has on one's mind and spirituality as well as on maintaining good energy flow through one's body. To use the hands to receive the energy and by-pass the head is to miss out on naturally improving one's growth and spirituality.

**The expansion of Eguchi's work**

Eguchi withdrew from the Gakkai after practicing Reiki for only two years. Once he started his own institute, several hundred people quickly became his students. This rapid growth alongside his lack of experience must have meant he had to go forward without solid foundations in his system.

One of the reasons it became so popular was an article published in a magazine in 1929 entitled, *Nihon oyobi Nihon-jin* (Japan and Japanese).

After that, a few hundred people a day would come to the institute. The article was written by the editor of the magazine and one of Eguchi's pupils, Koushi Mitsui. Mitsui was a literary man, a poet and a rightist (in Japan a rightist is someone who is nationalistic and believes the Emperor is God). He seems to be one of the key people characterizing Eguchi's therapy. His book, mentioned above, has been reprinted and when I read it, I felt very uncomfortable. He treats the hands-on therapy as *Shikisima no michi* (敷島の道 the way to ancient Japan) and thinks it is only for Japanese because the God energy comes through the Emperor. He believes Japanese people are exceptional and better than others.

Goro Miyazaki, the man who succeeded Eguchi's institute was also a poet, as was Kou Kijima, his successor. In their literature on the therapy they quote poems. It seems a little odd to practice a hands-on therapy in this way and make their passion for poetry necessary for everyone.

Eguchi's therapy eventually established its own breathing method, dietetics and other approaches not seen in Usui Reiki.

**Eguchi's message**

Despite the differences in Eguchi's therapy and my reservations about it, I would like to show the prospectus he wrote for his institute. Its composition is excellent and it is my favorite. In it, he describes the social situation at that time and I realized on reading it that it applies to present day society too.

Prospectus of Hands-on Institute by Toshihiro Eguchi

October 1928 (Showa 3)


New treatment methods become available one after another because of the new theories and new research techniques continually being developed by this scientific civilization. Some annoyingly propose medical treatments under the government or the separation of medicine and doctor's treatments. Still, we are seeing the sudden rise of new research in Chinese medicine and the growth of popularity of folk medicines. I think these rather prove there are still many significant problems in Western medical treatments.

There are yet a great number of middle to lower-class households that have no chance to benefit from modern medical treatments because the medical expenses are so heavy. Though this clearly indicates a need for many improvements and additions in the present organization for national medicare, it is never an easy task to correct such flaws in a system.

In recent years however, fortunately we have found an easy and reliable method to treat diseases. By applying one's hands on an affected area, various diseases can be cured. Human hands seem to have the ability to promote complete recovery from diseases much like a dog or cat cures an injury by licking. Curing diseases using one's hands has been performed since a long time ago, but often only by the spiritual power of an upstanding or saintly person, or by some miraculous ability acquired by a special ascetic. It has been performed only by a limited few but not by general households for everyday use.

As the age of science has come, hands-on therapies have been misunderstood as, or mixed up with, something superstitious. Intelligent people, especially, are apt to misunderstand and ignore hands-on therapies. Nevertheless, as we learned and tried the therapy we unexpectedly found that if a special method is applied once, to anyone, some power starts to radiate from the hands. This is an ability that humans naturally possess. The ability never ceases once activated. We found when a hand is applied to a problematic area of the body, the receiver's innate healing capacity is remarkably accelerated to cure diseases naturally. In addition, this therapy can be used quite safely even by a layman who has no anatomical knowledge because what he/she has to do is simply apply the hands quietly without giving any medicine or medical treatment. [Author's note: Eguchi does not use the word *Ki* (気) or energy. He uses *Chikara* (力) which means power.]

It means if this therapy is used alongside a medical diagnosis and treatment, combined as a nursing method, surprising effects can be seen. It is possible to activate the power from anyone's hands quite easily without exception. In most cases, a person can activate a useful amount of power if he/she practices for 30 to 40 minutes three days in a row. In this way, a single experienced teacher can activate 20 to 30 people at one time. By broadly spreading this hands-on therapy to each household, we would like to supplement the present medical care and at the same time to reduce the medical expenses in general households.

In addition to treating diseases, if this therapy became popular, it would bring psychological benefits, too. In this therapy a person places his/her hands directly on the client's body and stays there for a relatively long time, creating a sense of affinity between the client and the person treating. This is rarely found in medical care. When cured, a client seems to have deep gratitude.

Therefore, if this therapy was used among family members such as parent-child, wife-husband and brother-sister, it would naturally enrich their love and generate harmony among them. This therapy cultivates compassion by devoting one's precious time to helping and curing someone who suffers from a painful disease. People these days are apt to think that competing with each other is inevitable in order to make progress in life and society. Under these circumstances, where our society is becoming somewhat prosaic, spreading such a therapy is the best practical method for guiding our thought onto the right path.

Overwork and irritability are the common evils of modern culture. If family members healed each other with a heart-warming attitude, it would help to regain our original, Japanese, simple-mannered spirituality, contributing a great deal to people's lives.

Although there are dozens of hands-on therapies besides ours at the moment, some have stringent criteria to become members and some face difficult training in order to practice. The therapies of these groups would barely spread among general people. We therefore decided to introduce this therapy, with its unique simplicity and certainty, into each household.

I think Eguchi recognized the universality of human society quite well.

## Hands-on therapies used and originated by three Reijutsu-ka

As I mentioned before, in the Meiji, Taisho and early Showa eras (1870s-1930s) there were many Reijutsu-ka (miraculous method practitioners) who practiced various hand healing methods not related to Reiki. Since it would be difficult to describe all of them, I have studied three types and will explain a little about them.

1. *Tsunezo Ishi* (石井常造)
    - *Seiki Jikyou Ryoho* (生氣自強療法
       - Self-strengthening Therapy using Living Energy)
2. *Morihei Tanaka* (田中守平)
    - *Tairei-do* (太霊道 - Great Spiritual Way)
3. *Haruchika Noguchi* (野口晴哉)
    - *Yuki* (愉気 - Joyful Energy)

The best book on this subject, and the only one that thoroughly explains Reijutsu-ka is *Shin: Reijutsu-ka no Utage* (New: Feast of Miraculous Method Practitioners ISBN 488302248X) by *Hirotsugu Imura* (井村宏次)

though sadly it is currently only available in Japanese.

## 1. Tsunezo Ishii - Seiki Jikyou Ryoho (Self-Strengthening Therapy Using Living Energy)

Tsunezo Ishii was an elite, a major general in the Army. His book was published in 1927 (Showa 2), just one year after Usui died. His healing method, called Seiki Jikyo Ryoho has a resemblance to Reiki. Most of the hands-on therapies at that time were Qigong-like techniques - one of the most popular was *Reishi-jutsu* (霊子術) by Morihei Tanaka who I will talk about next. As far as I can tell from the literature on this and other popular methods, the energy they used was clearly not Reiki but Qigong, in which a therapist uses his/her own energy. However, Ishii's method did have some similarities to Reiki.

In Ishii's method, the practitioner improves his/her energy flow by doing a kind of stretching exercise called *Shinkei Kunren* (神経訓練 nerve training). This exercise is similar to that of Internal Qigong. Having performed the exercise, an energy starts to flow in various parts of the body. The therapist then sends this energy, called *Seiki* (生氣 living energy) to the client. Seiki generates involuntary body movements in the client which promotes the healing of diseases. This involuntary movement is similar to *Katsugen Undo* in Noguchi's therapy which I describe later.

Let's look at the nerve training exercise, how they used the living energy and the involuntary movements created in the client in a little more detail.

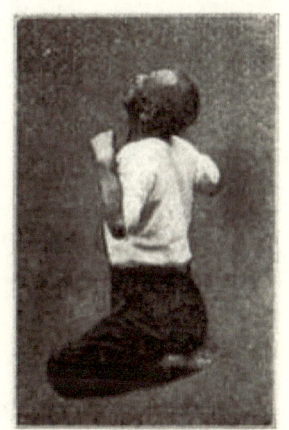

*a) Shinkei Kunren - nerve training*

In this exercise, one must use the posture shown in the photograph to train one's nerves, as they control various body functions according to Ishii. In his book, he illustrates a range of postures such as bending back one's spine, which is a common exercise. I tried this training for a few days but didn't feel any remarkable effects, though my body completely slackened after doing it. It should be noted that in Noguchi's bodywork, they use the same posture in order to promote involuntary movements, as described in his book, *Principles of a Healthy Life*.

*b) How to send Seiki - living energy*

In Ishii's therapy, once a practitioner has improved his or her energy flow by doing the nerve training, they can send Seiki (living energy) to a client. Though the nerve training is obviously not found in Reiki, his method for sending the energy is surprisingly similar to that of Usui Reiki.

Ishii's hands-on techniques are listed below:

- *Touching method* - the therapist applies the tips of three fingers together, just the thumb, or the middle finger. When an affected area is bigger, they use the whole hand, or both hands.
- *Rubbing method* - after applying a palm for a while, the therapist starts

rubbing and gradually increases the speed.

- *Patting method* - the therapist pats with his/her fingertips (four or five fingers), with the whole hand, or with a fist.
- *Fingertip without touch* - the therapist sends the energy from his/her fingertip(s) without touching the client.
- *Palm without touch* - the therapist sends the energy from his/her palm(s) without touching the client.
- *Send using the eyes* - Ishii says, "Seiki is expelled from various body parts···.enough energy can be sent simply by staring at an affected area."
- *Send using the mouth* - Ishii says, "Breathing means to exhale breath. The energy from the oral cavity is enhanced by exhaling breath. This method is suitable to use together with other methods."

If you know the techniques of Japanese Reiki, you'll be surprised to see that Ishii's method is almost identical to that of Japanese Reiki.

*c) Involuntary movements created by the living energy*
In contrast to Usui Reiki, Ishii's Seiki energy always induces involuntary movements in a clients body. According to Ishii, this movement is necessary to cure diseases. Ishii also describes a self-induction method to cause this movement in oneself. I tried it a few times but was not good at it. My body may not have been relaxed enough.

Incidentally, in Usui Reiki there is a method to make use of involuntary body movements. This is called *Reiki Undo* (霊気運動 Reiki movement or

Reiki exercise) which Frank Arjava Petter describes in detail on page 175 of *The Spirit of Reiki* (ISBN 0914955675). However, readers should know that this is not a traditional Reiki technique but one introduced by Koyama, the sixth president of the Gakkai in the 1970s, presumably as a replication of Noguchi's *Katsugen Undo*.

I have an article about Ishii posted on my Web site. His grandson found the article and visited me one day for a Reiki treatment. Unfortunately he has no memory of receiving Ishii's therapy but I was very grateful for his visit.

## 2. Morihei Tanaka - Taireido (The Great Spiritual Way)

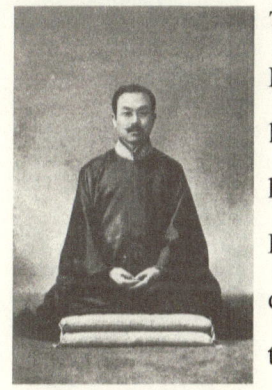

Taireido is a Qigong-like technique developed by Morihei Tanaka in the same era as Usui Reiki. His large organization had their own eschatology and held the belief that their god was above the Emperor. In this way they were in opposition with one of the most famous religious organizations at the time, Ohmoto-kyo. When they grew too large, the government cracked down on them.

I was introduced to two good books on Tanaka by one of my Jikiden Reiki colleagues. The first book is, *Lecture Notes on Taireido and Reishi Techniques* by Tanaka himself, and the second is, *Taireido: A Miraculous Method to Develop Supernatural Power* (ISBN: 4051034453) written by *Kazuyuki Takagi* (高木一行). These books gave me some insight into his techniques.

In the first half of his book, Tanaka describes his world view, which has similarities to a healthy spiritual way of thinking today. I resonated with his idea of *Zenshin* (全真 whole truth) which points to the fact that a truth can often change and is dependent on different conditions or different assumptions one may have. However, there is a truth beyond this idea of truth. For example, true happiness must incorporate both being happy and being unhappy, it is both bitter and sweet, death and life. Zenshin is the truth that integrates all.

In the chapter, *Universe*, he outlays his concepts of previous/next Universe and space time which are surprisingly quite consistent with modern cosmology while in the chapter *Society*, he considers our human society as a kind of living organism. I found I agreed with quite a few aspects of his thinking.

In the latter half of the book, he describes Reishi-jutsu (霊子術 miraculous element technique). To me, the relationship between his worldview and the technique is quite unclear. *There seems to be an unreasonable gap between his theory and practice.*

**My experience of Tanaka's miraculous element (Reishi) technique**

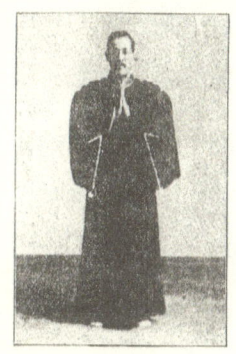 I have practiced Tanaka's *Standing Method to Induce Reishi Movement (Ritsu-shiki Reishi Kendo-ho* 立式霊子顕動法) several times. In this method, one applies strong force on both palms pressed together in front of one's chest as shown in the picture.

The first time I practiced, I felt energy as tingling and scratchy sensations in the center of my palms. It was so fascinating that I said, "Wow!" aloud. It didn't start any body movements but I became quite warm feeling the energy circulating and my hands became hot.

In Reiki when I practice Hatsurei-ho (発霊法 method to radiate Reiki) it usually takes 20-40 minutes to feel that amount of energy, but with this method it took only a minute. It was totally unexpected to me and I felt positive about this technique because of the clear feeling of the energy. I thought there was definitely something in it.

After practicing a few times, I started to feel my body moving, twitching oscillations not only in my arms but also deep in the core of my body. The Reishi movement (a clear cyclic oscillation) seemed to come when the oscillations became synchronized or coordinated together. I could feel slight vertical movements (縦動 *Tate do*) and horizontal movements (横動 *Yoko do*) but it is entirely possible I still might have been doing them consciously. I also felt the beginnings of jumping movements (跳動 *Hi do*).

71

If I had not been a Reiki practitioner and couldn't feel energy easily, I would have misunderstood those movements as exaggerated spasm-like movements that happen when one applies strong force on one's muscles. When I practiced this Kendo-Ho method, I felt energies were both oscillating and being amplified at the same time. I thought it was significant that a large amount of energy was generated.

Once I'd been practicing a while, even after taking a 20-30 minute rest, if I did Gassho (putting both palms together lightly) I could still feel small oscillations both in my hands and body. This stopped when I relaxed completely.

I felt very tired after doing this Kendo-Ho method. I would breathe intentionally for a while but still felt something strange. Perhaps if one practiced regularly it would all feel more natural? I'm not sure.

I would like to mention one more thing I found interesting.

One day, I was carrying a shoulder bag. My hand was on the strap while my arm was touching my chest. At some point I noticed that my hand and arm were warm. When I put more force on them I could clearly feel that more energy had accumulated. I guessed this happened because I was practicing Kendo-Ho at the time and so my muscles tended to generate the energy easily.

Despite my practice and the experiences I have related, I did not understand Tanaka's method for using the energy. I couldn't work out the relationship between the Kendo-Ho exercises he created and his *Sendo-Ho* (潜動 method for using energy). My experiment with Tanaka's Taireido ended at this point but I hope my experience gives some useful information to readers.

**A comparison of three energy techniques - Reiki, Qi-gong and Taireido**
One way to illustrate the difference between three energy techniques - Reiki, Qi-gong and Tanaka's Taireido - is to use the analogy of a heavy swing. Let's say the swing has to move to one side or the other to cause a flow of energy. The picture shows what you would need to do to initiate and maintain the flow using these three methods.

**Reiki**
Reiki is akin to simply leaning on the swing using natural bodyweight, producing a moderate constant current.

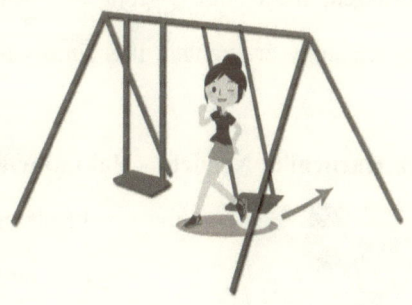

**Qi-gong**
Using Qi-gong to create the energy would be like using muscular power and sweating to push the swing in one direction.

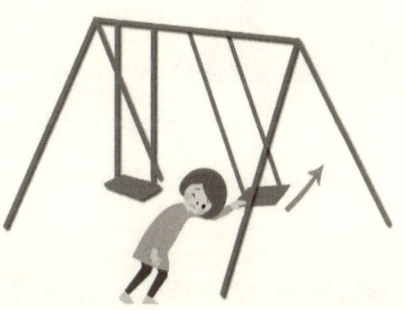

## Taireido - Kendo-Ho

This would be to keep increasing the amplitude of the swing by applying a small amount of muscular energy to the swing, moving in both directions, each time it swings. Because an oscillator can store energies, applying

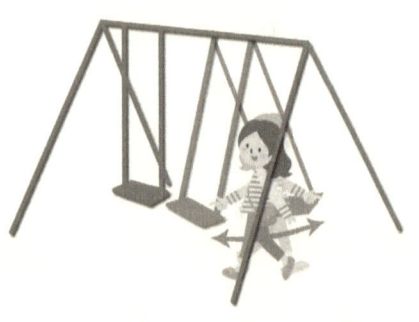

energy synchronously can increase the stored energy steadily resulting in a large amount of energy. Perhaps, if one used this method effectively one would be able to use a large amount of energy without such painful training or practice. I'm not sure.

As you can see, this comparison demonstrates clearly how Reiki is quite different from both Qi-gong and Taireido because it doesn't require one's own energy or strength, it is simply using one's natural weight.

## 3. Haruchika Noguchi - Yuki (Joyful Energy)

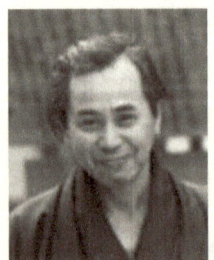

Yuki is a hands-on therapy. It's one of many techniques that Noguchi developed for his bodywork known as Noguchi Seitai. To discover more about Yuki and how it is different from Reiki I read the book, *Yuki Ho 1* (Yuki Method 1) which is not Noguchi's writing but a collection of his lectures and talks. The quotes below are from this book, available in Japanese only at http://www.zensei.co.jp/books/index.

*Yuki - How to Practice*

> "Yuki is done by inhaling into your lower abdomen then imagining exhaling from your hand(s) to send energy into a client's body" (page 42.)

> "Fill with energy by inhaling deeply into your abdomen and waist, focus your energy deep into the client's body, then exhale calmly with your hand(s) on the client" (page 192).

This basic method clearly indicates that Yuki is entirely different from Reiki. A Yuki practitioner has to maintain conscious breathing, inhaling and exhaling with great concentration. So Yuki is a Qi-gong-like technique rather than Reiki.

Doing this has adverse effects which I will mention later.

*Yuki - Initiation*

> "[Energy induction] Please sit in a circle. Connect to the person next to you by touching his/her wrist lightly. Close your eyes and just relax. The only thing you need to do is first synchronize your breath. It won't work if your breath is not synchronized. I will say, "Please inhale now." Inhale at the moment I finish saying, "now". After that, go back to normal breathing and relax with no facial expression. At the end, I will say "Please inhale now" again. Inhale together at that moment. That's all.

> "[Gassho for feeling the energy] Next, in front of your eyes, face your

palms towards each other with about a 3cm gap in between. If you keep staring at them, your palms slowly come to contact, then close your eyes. Inhale into your fingertips and exhale from your fingertips. Breathe imagining this and various things will happen to your hands.

"[Testing] Relax and point the fingertips of your right-hand toward the palm of your left-hand. After a while you will feel coolness, warmth or some other kind of sensation on your palm. Then move the fingertips around. The sensation will follow the movement" (page 64-65).

The initiation activates one's hands. Noguchi emphasizes synchronizing the breath. The initiation does not engage any part of the body other than the hands. As I mentioned in Eguchi's hands-on therapy, the critical difference between Reiki and other hands-on therapies is whether they flow energy through, and treat, one's head.

*Yuki - Mental Attitude*

"Without knowing what has changed, Yuki energy cheers up the client. It is not good for you to have an anxious or combative mind. A client recovers when you apply your hands with a natural and calm mind, which I call "Tenshin" (天心 heavenly mind)" (page 38).

"Tenshin is to rid yourself of all worldly thoughts and attain perfect serenity of mind. It is being open-minded and empty like the sky without any clouds. Even without confidence, if you do Yuki naturally with such a

> mind, it works naturally. It is not good to think or tell a client they will definitely recover based upon a few past experiences" (page 94).
>
> "While doing Yuki, I have no kind thoughts such as, 'I will make you live'. On the contrary, occasionally I even think 'You will die once you become old'" (page 41).

This Tenshin mind is similar to that in Reiki. The Yuki that Noguchi personally practiced probably contained a good amount of Reiki. However, it may be difficult to practice for a beginner or someone who can not establish Tenshin mind.

*Yuki - Reaction to the Energy*
Noguchi often uses the word, Kan-nou.

> "Kan-nou is the activation of the body's self-healing power as a reaction to the concentrated energy present when hands are applied. Kan-nou starts when the energy density becomes high enough through focusing your mind on an affected area (page 42).
>
> "You can not tell when you can finish Yuki in advance. You take off your hands when you feel a problem has gone after Kan-nou. Yuki is difficult to use for a professional practitioner" [Author's Note: because the therapy time is not predictable] (page 61).

In Reiki, we are unaware of Kan-nou because in Reiki Kan-nou happens all the time. As I mention later in 'Yuki - Problems', there are some cases where Kan-nou does not occur in Yuki. This may be the reason why Noguchi emphasizes Kan-nou.

*Yuki - Perceiving Sensations Similar to Byosen*

"If you have enough training to use the energy, your hand(s), when on an affected area can perceive some special sensations such as itching, a cool-wind, or warm feelings. You may occasionally feel pain or numbness. After some time, when the sensations go away and you feel normal, you may take your hand(s) off. In the hands-on therapy of Yuki, you need to concentrate the energy by keeping your hand(s) on until this Kan-nou completes" (page 193).

"Use Yuki on a part of the body that has become too sensitive due to excessive work. Apply your hand(s) on the area where you feel tingling or warm. Then, other parts that were idle or loosened start to generate tingling sensations. Move there and do Yuki. After that, other areas will start to generate coolness. Move and put your hand(s) on those areas. The body changes like this if you move around according to the change in sensation.

When you use Yuki, the client's body changes spontaneously. Your hands can move around by themselves without thinking. You do not have to search. I used to try to figure out the sequence of the changes, but recently I prefer to let my hands move by themselves to the next place" (page 164).

His descriptions of these are quite similar to Japanese Reiki. In Yuki, they feel sensations that are probably equivalent to byosen or hibiki. Noguchi also found a similar technique to *Reiji-ho* (霊示法 method of miraculous indication). In Reiji-ho, a practitioner intuitively lets their hands or intuition find a problem area. It is however, unknown how well practitioners other than Noguchi can use these techniques.

*Yuki - Problems*

I would like to bring attention to a couple of problems with Yuki that I observed when reading Noguchi's book.

"A father, whose son had difficulty in walking, was doing Yuki while anxious. The son became paralyzed when the father gave him Yuki. I said, "Stop. Your Yuki is anxious Yuki." His wife performed Yuki trying to make the son strong by any means but she was using struggling Yuki" (page 27).

"If you have a client who does not exhibit any Kan-nou at all, look for another practitioner. There are times where the energy is incompatible. The energy can be compatible or incompatible. The energy itself is neither good nor bad but it has compatibility. It is good to be compatible and bad to be incompatible" (page 70).

"I then started to teach Yuki to mothers who had children. Parents and their children exhibit Kan-nou most" (page 63).

> "Therefore, a practitioner should politely refuse an incompatible person rather than giving Yuki reluctantly" (page 109).

These are understandable consequences because a Yuki practitioner sends the energy intentionally, synchronizing with his/her breath. As a result, the intention of the practitioner tends to be mixed up with the energy. Although Noguchi himself is experienced enough to give positive energy, the parents in this first example inevitably had difficulty using Yuki because of how they were feeling.

It is also to be expected that a Yuki practitioner would come across incompatible clients because the energy they are giving to the client contains a substantial amount of the practitioner's personal energy. These are clear differences between Yuki and Reiki. Because the Reiki energy has no intention there can be no compatibility issue and the energy is not mixed with the practitioner's intentions or feelings.

*Yuki - Notable Observations*

*1. Yuki is not spontaneous and natural*

**If a person is relaxed and in a natural state, energy comes out spontaneously and naturally. That is Reiki.** Noguchi did not recognize this. He learned Reijutsu (a miraculous method) from *Doubetsu Matumoto* (松本道別) one of the Reijutsu practitioners, who developed a Qigong-like technique in which a practitioner sends energy with strong intentions. This may be the reason Noguchi was using his own energy and did not let go to allow Reiki to flow naturally.

## 2. No emphasis on energy coming through the head

One of the exceptional techniques in Reiki is to make careful use of one's head in an initiation (Reiju or attunement). Doing this generates a good energy flow through the body. In the case of Yuki, the intentional breath seems to supplement the energy, especially for beginners.

In addition, Reiki flowing through the head, both in an initiation and during treatment, contributes to one's spirituality. In Reiki, after one has received Reiju (attunement), Reiki flows through the head every time the person uses Reiki. The more one uses Reiki, the more one improves one's spirituality. The more a person's spirituality improves, the more Reiki flows.

## 3. Unwanted energy

As I've mentioned, the head is key during the Reiju that Usui established in order to increase the energy flow and contribute to spiritual growth. Yuki lacks this phenomenon, having practitioners use intentional breath instead. As a consequence, if they are sitting with unresolved anger or anxiety for example, it can result in unwanted energy being sent to the client or create the incompatibility issue Noguchi spoke of.

## Reiki is remarkable

In contrast to the other hands-on therapies, Japanese Reiki has a comprehensive framework with established techniques such as the basic hand usage, Gokai (Five Principles), Reiju (Attunement), Shirushi (Symbols), Kotodama (Word Spirit), Seiheki Chiryo (Mind-habit treatment), and Enkaku Chiryo (Distant healing). Furthermore, all these techniques are quite simple and easy to learn for everyone. Looking at these techniques, I sincerely recognize how great Usui was.

# Chapter 4  Usui Reiki Ryoho Gakkai

When Usui started his Reiki therapy in 1922, he soon established the Usui Reiki Ryoho Gakkai. The Japanese kanji for this is 臼井靈氣療法学会 where 臼井 is his name, 靈氣 is Reiki, 療法 is Ryoho which means therapy and 学会 is Gakkai meaning society.

The Gakkai has a history of more than 90 years and during those former years was supported by high-ranking naval officers. It had branches at most major naval ports such as Ohminato, Kure, Hiroshima and Saga. In 1930 it had about 7000 members according to the member list of that year. Some important members unfortunately withdrew from the Gakkai during the presidency of Juzaburo Ushida, the naval rear admiral who succeeded Usui as president in 1926.

Kaiji Tomita and Toshihiro Eguchi were two notable names who left and started their own hand healing groups as I mentioned in the last chapter. Another of those who withdrew, but continued with Usui's Reiki, was Chujiro Hayashi from whom the path to Western Reiki can be traced. Hayashi was one of the directors of the Gakkai, and despite the fact that most organizations are inflexible in one way or another, there must have been significant problems within the society if an important person such as Hayashi decided to withdraw. *Hiroshi Doi* (土居裕) author of, *A Modern Reiki Method for Healing* (ISBN 1886785333) surmises during an interview conducted by William Lee Rand that the reason Hayashi left, "...might be due to a conflict of opinion between him and the new president, Ushida."

The Gakkai consisted of various high-ranking people such as military officers, university professors, scholars, school teachers, company executives, politicians and often their wives. Out of twenty shihans (teachers) certified by Usui, about eight were naval officers, one was a school principal and one was a musician.

The Gakkai appears to be a very closed organization because there is no open information available from them. It has kept its doors securely closed to the general public since right after the war. There are probably a couple of reasons for this. Firstly, GHQ (the occupation headquarters in Japan) had purged all military personnel and were looking for possible war criminals among them and secondly, GHQ had banned alternative therapies (I go into this further in Chapter 8). Under such intimidating circumstances, many Gakkai members did not want to be exposed publicly. Hence, the Gakkai closed its doors firmly and shut out the public. It has remained that way since.

In *Okuzawa* adjacent to *Jiyugaoka* there used to be a naval village housing many high-ranking officers. Wanami, a vice-admiral and fifth president of the Gakkai lived in *Oyamadai* neighborhood of Jiyugaoka while the sixth president, Koyama lived in Jiyugaoka itself. One can speculate that they were giving professional Reiki treatments in this naval village but we can't know for sure.

What the Gakkai was doing after the war, and how it was doing it, is pretty much unknown territory. Foggy at best.

Koyama seems to have been very active in the Gakkai under the guidance of Wanami before she became president. It appears that many clients visited her for Reiki treatments and that she gave distant healings. There are more details on this in Chapter 6.

Currently, the Gakkai has a regulation that they can only use Reiki on other Gakkai members or their families. It is possible to treat a member of the public not involved with the society, but the Gakkai member needs a license issued by the president to do so. One can become a member of the Gakkai only through a formal introduction by an existing member. There is no open literature or printed materials, no internet site or contact address, which is extremely unusual in this age of information! The sole public record of their existence is a registered trademark no.4466242 Shinshin Kaizen Usui Reiki Ryoho Gakkai.

I believe it is praiseworthy that the Gakkai was kept alive even when facing severe difficulties during and after the war. Nevertheless, seeing that they remain closed today, they seem to have been left behind the times somewhat. In contrast with the period of occupation when Western medical care was compulsory, many alternative therapies are now recognized, practiced and genuinely helpful in people's daily lives.

Since the 80s and 90s these therapies have been practiced in a *grey zone* where they are not permitted to refer to what they do as *treatments*. Even without this institutional support, many practitioners and therapists had the courage to, and continue to, provide effective therapies publicly.

The Gakkai continues to claim that they cannot be open because traditional Reiki is deemed a quasi-medical treatment, but this seems like a poor excuse to me. The members of *Jikiden Reiki* (直傳靈氣) another traditional Reiki group in Japan are successfully providing Reiki as an alternative therapy in such a grey zone. They are demonstrating that if one has the will, it is possible to openly use Reiki as an effective therapy without help from the establishment. By keeping Reiki under wraps, the Gakkai almost appear to look down on it, reducing it to merely a hobby for the members.

When Usui started Reiki, his aspiration was that it be used to help large numbers of ordinary people. Even though he did not allow commercial advertising, the membership of the Gakkai increased from 2,000 in 1926 to around 7,000 by 1930 and we know that he was treating the general public because of his actions after the Great Kanto Earthquake. However, after the war, the Gakkai lost such momentum that the numbers have now decreased to only a few hundred.

## Chapter 5   Chujiro Hayashi

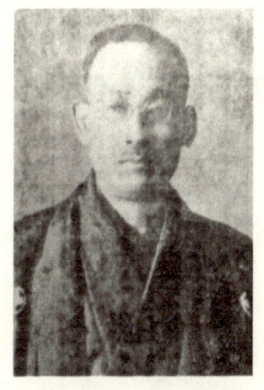 Chujiro Hayashi (1879-1940) was born in Kanagawa and graduated from the 30th graduating class of the Naval Academy in 1902 at age 23. After retiring from the Navy at 47 years old, Hayashi started his own Reiki center in Shinano-machi.

The Reiki center had a relatively large staff with 16 therapists. To have a clinic providing Reiki treatments on such a scale today is unimaginable. I would love to transport myself through time to see Hayashi's clinic for myself and to witness Reiki being used in such a medical setting. I'd love to join them in giving Reiki! The social systems back then may have been old-fashioned but it has to be said some things in the past seem to be more advanced, or at least more innovative.

It is not confirmed that Hayashi was a certified doctor. However, the official tax payment record for Hayashi lists his occupation as a doctor. The document was found at the National Diet Library after the person who found it had thoroughly investigated the taxpayer records of the citizens of Tokyo in prewar years. The document for Hayashi is registered under the same address as Hayashi's Reiki center.

Chujiro Hayashi contributed significantly to the spread of Reiki, and reached a much wider population than the Gakkai. He trained Hawayo Takata, a second generation Japanese American lady living in Hawaii. It was through her that Reiki spread to the West. He visited Hawaii to help Takata in spreading Reiki and taught the students who started Jikiden Reiki in Japan, which follows Hayashi's teachings from those days. Jikiden Reiki is believed to be the only system in the world today that teaches authentic Japanese Reiki to anyone who wishes to learn. You can learn more about this at http://www.jikiden-reiki.com.

After Hayashi passed away in 1940, his wife, Chie Hayashi succeeded his institute. According to the member list of the Gakkai in the year 1928, Chie was a registered member. Following her husband's death she continued to work with Reiki, however, some years after the war finished, she became a devout follower of a religion known today as *Soka Gakkai* (創価学会). The kanji characters for Soka Gakkai are: 創: to create, creation; 価: values; 学会: institute, society.

At the time Chie Hayashi joined, they were only a small group of fewer than 1000 people and were an educational group who studied Buddhism. After the postwar GHQ occupation, they became a religious organization and grew rapidly. According to their website the number of households in Japan today with residents who are members of Soka Gakkai is 8,270,000. They control the political party, *KoumeiToh* (公明党).

Chie's affiliation with this religion made her students feel uncomfortable and many left the Hayashi Reiki Institute. In the book, *The Hayashi Reiki Manual* by Frank Arjava Petter and Tadao Yamaguchi you can find the address of the Hayashi Reiki Center on page 13. In Hayashi's time it was 28 Higashi Shinano-machi, Yotsuya-ward, Tokyo but today it is 27 Shinano-machi, Shinjuku-ward, Tokyo. Chie donated the land owned by the Hayashi Reiki Institute to the Soka Gakkai and today a large group of their buildings are there.

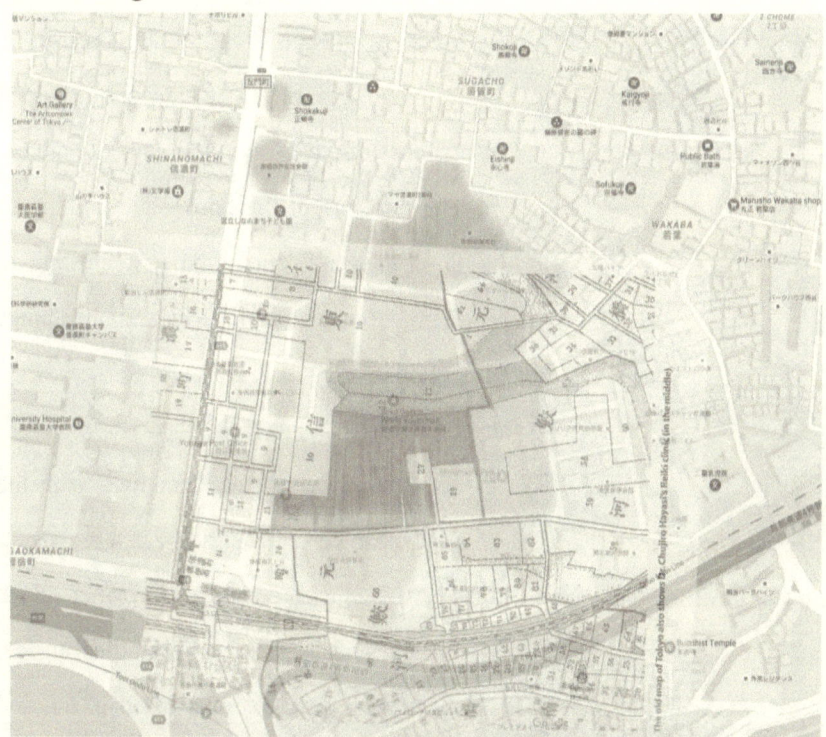

The above map shows the Soka Gakkai headquarters today. The present Soka Gakkai property is light blue and has been underlaid beneath the old map found by Frank Arjava Petter where Hayashi's address is marked as a dark grey area at the center. As you can see, Soka Gakkai now occupy a huge area of approximately 300 × 500m centered at the former Hayashi's clinic.

Please note that this religious institute has nothing whatsoever to do with Reiki.

## Other points of interest concerning Hayashi

*Naval maintenance manual*

I have found a book I am 90% sure was written by Chujiro Hayashi. It is not a general publication but a manual for the maintenance of equipment

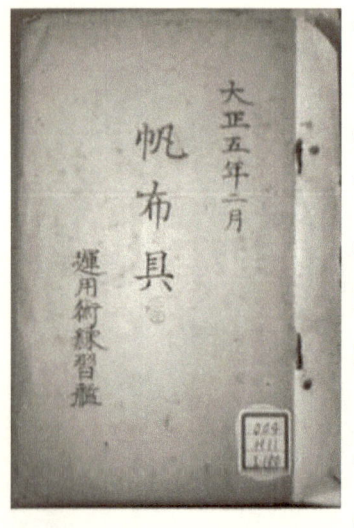

on a naval operation training vessel. A training vessel is a decommissioned sailboat used in the training of sailors. The contents of the book have nothing to do with Reiki, but I find it interesting to learn more about Hayashi and the things he did.

The manual is about 20cm long with the pages stapled together and has a red stamp on the cover saying, *Ishida* (石田), who must have been the owner of the

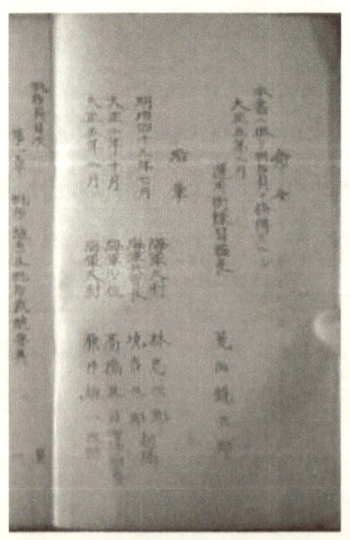

manual and used it for his studies. Inside, there are a few notes scrawled in ink and various corrections of numbers and words written as a student would when being taught in class, but it is quite well-preserved. Please note when looking at the photographs that the Japanese language is written vertically from top to bottom with columns read from right to left.

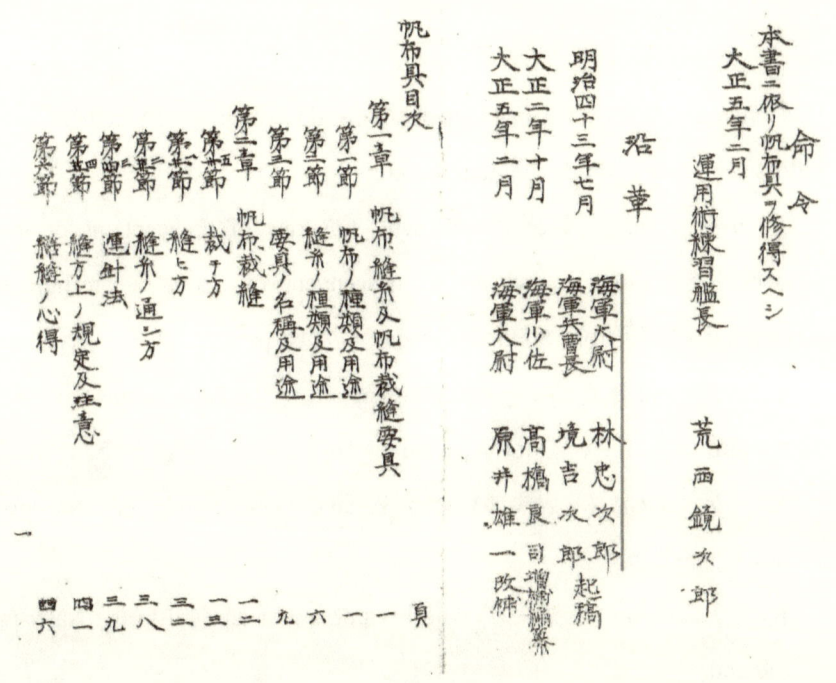

命令

本書ニ依リ帆布具ヲ修得スヘシ

大正五年二月

運用術練習艦長　　荒西鏡次郎

沿革

明治四十三年七月　海軍大尉　林忠次郎　起稿
大正二年十月　　　海軍兵曹長　境吉次郎
大正五年二月　　　海軍少佐　髙橋良
　　　　　　　　　海軍大尉　原井雄一　改補

On the back cover you can see a name assumed to be Hayashi (林忠次郎), author of the first edition in 1910 (明治 四十三年). His title is lieutenant in the Navy (海軍大尉). Hayashi was 31 years old in 1910. It makes sense chronologically that he would be a lieutenant if he was a captain by age of 47 when he retired from the Navy. The naval ranks he would have gone through are:

→ warrant officer

→ ensign

→ sub-lieutenant

→ lieutenant

→ lieutenant commander

→ commander

→ captain

This photograph shows a page in the book documenting the authors and editors. The names on the photograph are:

- *Kyojiro Aranishi* (荒西鏡次郎) who was one of the captains of the operation training vessel and a descendent of Soma, a prestigious samurai family from Shimousa (today's Chiba prefecture). He served as a rear general in the Navy and then captain of the Navy battleship Fuji.
- Chujiro Hayashi (林忠次郎) [at the marker]
- *Kichijiro Sakai* (境吉次郎) who I have been unable to find any information on.
- *Ryoji Takahashi* (髙橋良司) who became a rear admiral in the Navy in the end.
- *Yuichiro Harui* (原井雄一) from Hiroshima who was lieutenant when the book was written and later became a lieutenant commander.

I found the booklet in the Tokyo University of Marine Science and Technology but it originally came from the library of Dr. *Yukichi Habara* (羽原又吉 1882〜1969) who was a researcher of fishery. I have no idea how this manual came to be in his possession but Dr. Habara must have acquired it through someone else as it was a confidential manual for Navy personnel only and he was not a naval man. Fortunately, it had found its way to a civilian's bookshelf by chance. Interestingly, Dr Habara passed away at an address registered to Ishida in Oita prefecture, so I suspect it is related to the Ishida who originally owned the manual.

This booklet doesn't offer any new information regarding Reiki and there is no way to prove this manual was written by our Hayashi, but due to the fact that there is no record of another Chujiro Hayashi in the Navy in those days, I feel certain it is him.

Various documents and items of information on *the Japanese Navy are available on the database of the Japan Center for Asian Historic Records / National Archives of Japan* at http://www.jacar.go.jp/. On this site, you can find several documents under the name, Chujiro Hayashi, though I did not find anything important.

*Cherry-blossom viewing*

In some official documents of the naval ministry, I came across the lists of participants in some traditional Japanese seasonal events such as cherry-blossom viewing and chrysanthemum viewing.

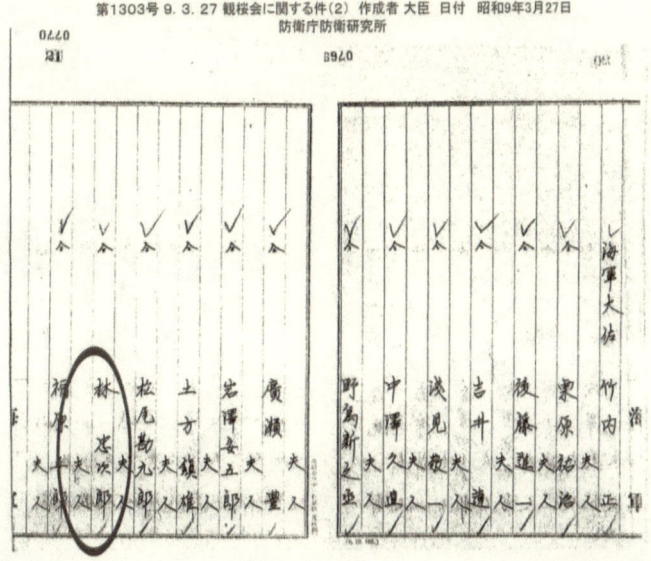

第1303号 9.3.27 観桜会に関する件(2) 作成者 大臣 日付 昭和9年3月27日
防衛庁防衛研究所

The photograph in the previous page shows the list for a cherry-blossom viewing event that took place in 1934. The marker shows that Hayashi 林 忠次郎 and his wife, listed as 夫人, were participants of the event. This information is not useful in terms of Reiki knowledge but going through all the documents available at random is the only way to find useful ones. Searching for information using the words *Reiki and Hayashi* has not brought anything up. I didn't find anything of significance when searching the names of other Gakkai members who were officers in the Navy either. The documents I'm speaking of exist in the database of *the National Institute for Defense Studies* at http://www.nids.go.jp/ and you are welcome to access them there.

Perhaps in the future we will find more information on the life of Chujiro Hayashi, but for now it is enough to appreciate his achievements and acknowledge that both Reiki in the West and Japanese Reiki in Japan are alive today thanks to him.

# Chapter 6    Past Meets Present

Running a Reiki school and therapy center gives me the chance to meet people from a wide variety of backgrounds. Occasionally, I come across people whose relatives practiced hands-on therapies or traditional Reiki during the prewar period. These people have generously related stories about their relatives and I'd like to share some of their precious experiences with you here, taking care not to encroach on their privacy.

## Case A - A lady whose grandmother was using Reiki

*Ms A's grandmother used Reiki until she passed away in 1999. She talked to me about her.*

In 1934, her son contracted peritonitis and had a high fever as a result. She took him to a clinic to treat the problem and while she was there a nurse told her about Reiki. Subsequently, she took her son to receive Reiki from Ms *Tose Endo* in *Zoshigaya*, Tokyo, and the boy recovered well as a result. Ms A's grandmother told her that Tose Endo had learned Reiki from a teacher named ***Jujiro Hayashi*** who had a Reiki therapy center until 1940. This must have been Chujiro Hayashi.

The grandmother learned Reiki with Tose Endo and used it alongside homeopathy, which was an innovative approach to health and healing in prewar Japan. She could be said to be a pioneer of complementary medicine in those days.

Ms A received Reiju (attunements) from her grandmother and has been using Reiki since then. Here is a surviving lineage from Hayashi.

Hayashi → Tose Endo → Ms A's grandmother → Ms A.

However, as far as I could tell from our conversation, her grandmother didn't teach her any Shirushi (symbols), Jumon, Ketsueki-Kokan ho, Byosen, or how to do Reiju. She had not heard of the Gokai either.

Information on students of Hayashi is scarce and aside from the Yamaguchis of Jikiden Reiki, this is the only one I am aware of.

## Case B - A grandmother practicing Reiki for a living

*Ms B's grandmother, a former nurse who also passed away in 1999, practiced Reiki for a living.*

She learned Reiki from a teacher named *Kuroda*, who was about 30 years old at the time and lived in a suburb of Tokyo - either *Nakano* or *Suginami*. After learning, she would regularly attend follow-up meetings and her daughter, Ms B's mother, often went along.

During the war, Ms B's grandmother was evacuated to *Hokkaido*, a northern island of Japan. After the war, she returned to Tokyo and continued her profession as a full time Reiki practitioner until 1959. She had a huge number of clients, sometimes so many that she would treat two clients simultaneously, placing one hand on each client while others would be waiting in the lobby for their treatments. Even though the number of people she treated decreased as she became older, she continued to practice Reiki until the last moments of her life.

This lady used the term, *Reiki o kakeru*, meaning, *to give Reiki*. This is the same phrase the Yamaguchis of Jikiden Reiki use. There are many ways to express 'to give Reiki' in Japanese. Usually, people say, Reiki o okuru (send Reiki), Reiki o suru (do Reiki) or Reiki o tsukau (use Reiki). The Yamaguchis use, Reiki o kakeru (pour Reiki) which may well be a particular expression that Hayashi used, though we can't be sure. As Ms B's grandmother used the same unusual expression she could well have learned Reiki from a teacher of Hayashi's lineage.

Ms B never heard her grandmother mention the words Reiju, Gokai or Byosen and is not sure she ever practiced distant healing. Her grandmother did however, sometimes hold free classes to teach Reiki to her clients and encouraged them to use it to help their families.

Ms B has taken a Jikiden Reiki course and when she returned home and performed the Ketsueki-Kokan ho (blood circulation method) on her relatives, she was surprised to hear them say, "I know this! Grandma did this for me before!" The grandmother's Reiki from all that time ago had come back into their lives today.

## Case C - A grandfather practicing Teate-Ryoji

*Ms C's grandfather used to practice the hands-on therapy known as Teate Ryoji*, founded by Toshitaka Eguchi. Eguchi belonged to the Gakkai for two years and I have explained a little about him and the therapy he developed in Chapter 3.

Ms C was one of my Jikiden Reiki students who has become a shihan (teacher) and actively promotes Reiki. She doesn't remember much about how her grandfather treated people with Eguchi's method.

It is interesting to note that it is not unusual to find a student in my class whose grandparent used to practice these kinds of hands-on healings or religious hand-healing such as Tenri-kyo (天理教, the Tenri sect). These students have only vague memories of receiving healing during their childhood or seeing family members receive it. However, unlike Reiki, I have not encountered any cases in which the religious healing methods were handed down to their children or grandchildren.

## Case D   A member of the Gakkai

*Ms D was a member of the Usui Reiki Ryoho Gakkai during the 1980s.*

I was interested in how she came to be a member. She told me that she had been hospitalized and formed a friendship with a lady in the hospital. One day when they were chatting this lady told her that though it may be difficult to believe, there was something called Reiki that would heal her son's asthma. She kindly introduced Ms D to Koyama of the Gakkai. Her son went once a week to receive treatments with Koyama, the president of the Gakkai at the time. She was impressed with Koyama's enthusiasm and recalls how attentively she treated her son who was so young that he couldn't stay still during the treatments. Sometimes Koyama switched from hands-on to hands-over his body if he was moving too much. As far as she can remember, the fee for one session was 1,000 yen which is about 10 US dollars in the current exchange rate.

Ms D became a member of the Gakkai herself and learned Reiki as Koyama had suggested. The Gakkai must have been more flexible and open than it is now if a usual member of the public was able to join.

Ms D doesn't remember how the Reiju was conducted or the contents of the class. This may be because the very first class given by the Gakkai and Hayashi (called the sixth grade) didn't give Reiju, it was only lectures. Or, as it was 20 years since she had trained when I interviewed her, she may simply not be able to remember. She did mention though, that she was told to practice *Ken-Yoku* (乾浴, dry-bathing technique) before using Reiki, which she found tiresome when she came to do treatments. Ken-yoku was not taught in Hayashi's lineage.

When recalling her experience of participating in Gakkai workshops in those days, Ms D says Koyama told participants to bring a photo of a family member or a friend. She would perform distant Reiki by holding each photo, one by one, in her hand while talking and teaching the class.

On another occasion, Ms D took her child to a Gakkai meeting. The child had a fever at the time and afterwards, Koyama came to her and told her she had been sending distant Reiki to her during the meeting. By the time they arrived home, her child's fever had gone down.

I am very impressed with Koyama's passion in using Reiki in such ways, which is something we must all learn. The Gakkai use the expression *o-Reiki* instead of just Reiki, where the o- is polite and indicates deep respect in Japanese. This illustrates how highly it is regarded by them.

Sadly, Ms D was never confident in using Reiki so she gradually lost interest and faded away from the Gakkai gatherings. They did not seem to place great importance on seminars in the Gakkai, perhaps believing that Reiki would require gradual long-term learning. It's probable that they left it up to the motivation of each member to deepen their learning.

## Case E - An acquaintance of Koyama

Ms E was acquainted with Koyama's family. I had the chance to meet her and asked her what Koyama was like. She told me many stories about her though I will only share the ones that maintain the privacy of the family.

Ms E's grandmother was an active member of the Gakkai. Often, when she went to visit her grandmother as a child, she wasn't home. She was told her grandmother, *'went out for Reiki'*.

The session fee, she remembers, was 1,000 yen in the days of Koyama, which is the same fee mentioned in Case D. They would usually give Reiki to a client who was sitting on a chair. In some cases they used a cotton towel to cover the head and lay their hands over it on the forehead and the back of the head. When they had many clients, Koyama's students began the treatments and Koyama finished up the sessions. For these multiple treatments there would be several chairs placed in the treatment room.

In other stories Ms E recounted, Koyama gave Reiju to a handkerchief or a crystal for people to keep as a talisman (they give Reiju to crystals in Jikiden Reiki too). Ms E had a handkerchief that had been given Reiju and kept it in her school bag. She recalls her father carrying one too and believes he escaped a plane crash that occurred in the waters close to *Haneda*, Tokyo in 1966 because of it. Miraculously, he had to change his flight at the last minute. All 133 passengers aboard the plane he was supposed to take were killed.

Koyama's husband was a scholar and another lady brought for treatments by Koyama was married to a scholar. He was teaching some of the imperial family. Everything I've heard about these kinds of things has made me realize that the Gakkai had a great many connections to people from the upper ranges of society.

### Important roles played by women

The above cases provide rare and precious links from the past to the present, told through the stories of five women. I will talk more about the important role of women in Reiki in Chapter 9 when I discuss Hawayo Takata. However I'd like to bring attention now to the fact that several women, including Takata, Chiyoko Yamaguchi of Jikiden Reiki and others, played leading roles in handing Reiki down to later generations. I must admit that women have more patient and persistent characteristics than men do. It is very intriguing and admirable to me.

# Chapter 7   Reiki and The Road to War

The war had a significant impact on Reiki practitioners because of connections with the Navy, which openly acknowledged Reiki. Several of the Usui Reiki Ryoho Gakkai representatives were in the Navy, quite a few Navy officials were shihans and Hayashi himself was a Navy captain.

## Hayashi's dilemma

Through his Japanese Hawaiian student, Hawayo Takata, Hayashi had the opportunity to teach Reiki in Hawaii. He travelled there in October 1937 and stayed five months, leaving in February 1938 according to his farewell speech published in the Hawaii Hochi newspaper. He gave 14 seminars and 350 people became members of his institute during his time there. (The detail report on his visit to Hawaii is shown in http://jikiden-reiki-nishina.com/hawaii/.)

Hawaii, home to a US Naval Pacific Fleet port at the time, was of high strategic importance. Being located between mainland US and Japan, it was a geographically advantageous spot for the military to control. Both countries knew what was likely to come, Hawaii was a prime target for Japan should they choose to go to war with the US. The US Army started restrictions on Japanese activities in Hawaii from the mid to late 1930s and in 1940 the US Army, FBI and local police made plans to arrest and confine influential Japanese citizens there. Japan meanwhile, had been looking at the potential advantage of an attack on Hawaii since 1928 and seriously considered an air strike as early as January 1941. Both sides were preparing.

This development was very challenging for Hayashi. Imagine how agonizing it must have been for him to learn that Hawaii, where he had so many students, was about to be attacked. The place he had made such an effort to spread Reiki would be turned into a horrific battle scene by the Japanese Navy - the Navy he belonged to. A naval attack on Hawaii would be a terrible betrayal to Takata and the people he met and taught there. It makes my heart ache to imagine how he must have felt.

It is known that Hayashi committed suicide in 1940. It may well have been because he could not face the the seemingly impossible situation with Reiki, his naval duties and the coming war in Hawaii.

Another viewpoint proposes that because of his connection to the area, Hayashi may have been given the naval mission of spying in Hawaii, which he avoided by killing himself. Regardless, we can be sure that his act of bringing Reiki from Japan to Hawaii, though it may well have cost him his life, was what led to the spread of Reiki to the West.

**Major events as Japan rushed headlong down the road to war**
- Japanese military action abroad is preceded by ○
- Japanese domestic laws and events are preceded by ◎
- Other countries' military action is preceded by ◇

○ Sep. 18, 1931 Outbreak of the *Manchurian Incident* - pretext for the

Japanese invasion of northeastern China in the same year.

○ Feb.26, 1936 *The February 26 Incident* (known as the 2.26 Incident) - an attempted coup d'etat in Japan. It was organized by a group of young Japanese Army officers with the goal of purging the government and military leadership of their factional rivals and ideological opponents.

○ Jul. 7, 1937 *Sino-Japanese War* (1937-45) erupts.

○ Feb. 13, 1937 *Japanese Army occupies Nanking*, China.

● Oct. 1937 - Feb. 1938 *Hayashi's visit to Hawaii*

◎ Apr. 1, 1938 *National General Mobilization Law* issued to allow use of civilian resources for war

◎ Apr. 5, 1939 Law to *control contents of movies.*

◎ Jun. 16, 1939 Neon *advertisements* and *hair perms banned.*

◇ Sep. 1, 1939 *German Air force/Army invades Poland* (Outbreak of WW2).

◎ Oct.18, 1939 *Japanese government freezes price of commodities and wages.*

◎ Feb.13, 1940 *Rice distribution under the food-control system* starts.

◇ May 10, 1940 *German Army bombs Benelux* (Belgium, the Netherlands and Luxembourg).

● May 11, 1940 *Chujiro Hayashi passes away.*

◎ Jun. 1, 1940 *Sugar and matches* become items to be delivered through the *ration system.*

◇ Jun. 3, 1940 *German Air Force bombs Paris.*

◇ Jun. 10, 1940 *Italy declares war against England and France.*

◎ Jul. 7, 1940 *Restriction on selling luxury products* starts.

◎ Aug. 1, 1940 *Serving rice* in Tokyo restaurants banned, restricted selling time of rice.

◎ Aug. 8, 1940 *Flour distribution under the food-control system* starts.

○ Sep. 23, 1940 *Japanese Army occupies Northern French Indo-China.*

○ Sep. 27, 1940 *Japan enters into a triple alliance with Germany and Italy.*

◎ Oct. 12, 1940 *Imperial Rule Assistance* Association formed.

◎ Nov. 2, 1940 Imperial ordinance to *encourage people to wear national clothing.*

◎ Dec.12, 1940 Cabinet Information Board established for *control of free speech and public opinion.*


The wartime regime in Japan was established by *Fumimaro Konoe*'s government in 1940. Restrictions on speech and other daily activities came into play as well as psychological influence through mottos such as *Luxury is an Enemy.*

In Europe, Germany and Italy were already engaged in war with England and France. Japan allied with the former while the US was allied with the latter. War between the two countries was imminent.


○ Jul. 1941 *Japan invades Southern French Indo-China.*

◎ Oct. 1941 *Inauguration of the Cabinet of Hideki Tojo* (military cabinet).

○ Dec. 8, 1941 *Japanese Navy attacks Pearl Harbor* (Pacific War).


The *2.26 Incident* in 1936 by part of the Army led to a conservative swing in Japanese politics. The Army expanded the War in China and advocated war with the US, while the Navy took a stand against the war. Naval Commander Isoroku Yamamoto was tenaciously opposed to starting a war with the US. Yet it is a sad irony in history that it was Commander Yamamoto himself who drew up the plan to attack Pearl Harbor and directed the action. Having been so opposed to the war, he turned out to be the one to initiate it. This shows the serious problem in the decision making processes of the Japanese government in those days.

Mar. 10 1945 Indiscriminate *bombing on Tokyo city by US.*

Apr. - Jun. 1945 *US invades Okinawa.*

Jul. 26, 1945 US, UK and China *demands Japan's unconditional surrender.*

Aug. 6, 1945 *Atomic bombing of Hiroshima by US.*

Aug. 8, 1945 *The Soviet Union declares war on Japan.*

Aug. 9, 1945 *Atomic bombing of Nagasaki by US.*

Aug.15, 1945 *Japan surrenders to the Allied Nations.*

**Takata's dilemma**

Hearing of the death of her beloved teacher, Hayashi, must have deeply affected Takata, but that was just the beginning of an intensely difficult time for her. Takata had to go through the agonizing experience of watching the Japanese Navy, so closely associated with Reiki, attack her homeland. By then, she had helped a great many people with the Reiki she had learned from a Japanese officer in the Navy, the same Navy that was now killing her fellow Hawaiians. Her dilemma is beyond imagination. I have not found any useful information on how she lived and what she went through emotionally during the war. All we can do is guess as to what it was like for her.

Most people would have given up on Reiki under these circumstances. The Americans continued actively stirring up the spirit of war among the people of Hawaii with slogans such as, *Remember Pearl Harbor*. If she had emphasized Reiki as being a therapy from Japan she would have come across severe criticism, even hatred from almost everyone around her. However, she continued her Reiki activities in Hawaii and I'll look at these in more depth in Chapter 9.

Her tenacity in the face of such extreme challenges illustrates her great trust in Reiki. Of course it was the truth and power of Reiki that prompted her to continue but *without her great energy to endure so many trials and tribulations in promoting it, we could well have lost Reiki today*.

# Chapter 8   Postwar Japan under Occupation

Roughly two million Japanese military personnel and 700,000 Japanese civilians died during the Pacific War between 1941 and 1945. 19 million non-Japanese, of which about half were Chinese, died in the fight against Japan. Today, these figures are far beyond our imagination and although the exact numbers are arguable, it is undeniable that the peace we enjoy today is based on the sacrifice of innumerable lives. Such a death toll suggests that things were to change drastically after the war. There were indeed a great many changes.

You may wonder why hands-on therapies such as Reiki declined after the war in Japan. I can see many reasons why this happened. People's mentality changed drastically during the Allied occupation, mostly due to GHQ (General Headquarters of the Allied Forces) policy. Anything scientifically inexplicable became seen as untrustworthy or strange and traditional Japanese values declined. Alongside the GHQ policies, people began to look at mistakes made during the war and as it turned out, it wasn't just the Japanese military who had been defeated, the country had faced cultural defeat as well.

Let's look at what happened in Japan after the war and how it changed the way people thought.

**Health and social changes made by GHQ during the occupation**

Japan experienced a sudden change in social conditions as a result of the occupation by the Allies, led by the United States of America. GHQ executed massive transformation across all sectors of society with the aim of preventing Japan from ever being in a position to stand against the US again. There were, however, members of GHQ who wanted to approach the reformation with some degree of benevolence.

GHQ took control by issuing, 'Supreme Commander for the Allied Powers Directives' (SCAPIN). They first cracked down on anything military and issued purge directives. In January 1946, SCAPIN 550 and 560 ordered the, 'Removal and Exclusion of Undesirable Personnel from Public Office'. Of those purged from public service, about 80 percent were Army and Naval personnel, the number totaling 167,035 (Masanori Nakamura *Occupation and reform* 占領と改革 ISBN 400003684X). At the same time, GHQ was searching for war criminals among politicians and military personnel. These must have dealt quite a blow to the Usui Reiki Ryoho Gakkai as some were military personnel and they kept a close relationship with the Navy.

In addition, anything seeming remotely 'military' to Americans was also banned. This included martial arts such as *Judo* (柔道), *Karate* (空手), *Kendo* (剣道), *Kyudo* (弓道 archery), and even *Sado* (茶道 tea ceremony) as well as historical plays, *Kabuki* (歌舞伎) and Shinto rituals. Under such circumstances, members of the Gakkai must have felt it dangerous to continue their activities because many of them were of a high social status.

During this time, Japan was virtually in ruins as a result of repeated bombing by the US Air Force on a number of cities. Social infrastructure had been destroyed and the number of war orphans was on the rise. Medical and hygiene standards, already significantly below the US in prewar times, were in decline. This, coupled with the chaos and poverty caused by war and air strikes, led to a high infant mortality rate and the constant threat of epidemics such as smallpox, cholera, dysentery, venereal disease, polio, Japanese encephalitis and tuberculosis.

Under such circumstances, GHQ conducted large-scale reformation in the field of medicine and hygiene under the command of Brigadier General Crawford F. Sams. They expanded public health facilities across the board, conducting such things as tap water chlorination and DDT spraying. GHQ also aimed to improve child nutrition, resuming school lunch programs with an emphasis on protein intake. These policies by General Sams undeniably saved many Japanese. (Crawford F. Sams *DDT Revolution* DDT革命 ISBN 4000014455, nearly identical to Crawford F. Sams *Medic: The Mission of an American Military Doctor in Occupied Japan and Wartorn Korea* ISBN 0765600307, but some data has been corrected in the Japanese edition.)

Educational movies were created to spread greater hygiene awareness. Traditional Japanese ways of treating illness such as the incantations and prayers used in Shinto and Shugendo were criticized in these movies. Americans of that time would have considered these folk and home remedies to be superstitious and primitive, especially when practiced in a country with so little awareness of hygiene. There is an interesting description by General Sams on page 255 of his book *DDT Revolution* that indicates how the practice of moxa cautery (the burning of mugwort on particular points of the body, often used alongside acupuncture) was mistaken for torture:

> "This therapy had been applied to the affected area on a captured American soldier. As a result, the captive reported upon release that he had been tortured in prison....... A prosecutor once came to visit me seeking an indictment of the Japanese doctor as a war criminal on the grounds of using acupuncture and moxa cautery on US captives."

General Sams talked further on the issue of traditional Japanese medicine in the same literature (pp.255-6):

> "All countries, including the US have the problem of quasi-medical practice. ....we investigated the social status of those people engaged in these quasi-medical practices. A certain very interesting political battle was triggered during the process. We came to realize that the practice of acupuncture had been accepted as a privilege for visually impaired people. If we enact license laws to ban acupuncture we will thereby deprive them of their privilege, removing the livelihood of all the visually impaired people in Japan. Such a dilemma is..."

This gives some insight into how General Sams viewed these therapies. Despite his careful consideration here, he refers to them as quasi-medical.

Since such therapies were undefined and unclear in their effect, they were thought to interfere with the introduction of advanced medical technology by GHQ. The terms, 'alternative therapy' or 'complementary therapy' didn't exist then and the New Age movement was to come much later. At that time, scientism was predominant in the US. In fact, it was science and technology that had led the Allies to victory through the development and production of the atomic bombs.

Consequently, GHQ banned the practice of folk remedies and traditional therapies. There were a few exceptions made thanks to the efforts of those who managed to convince GHQ of their efficacy. The law, issued in 1947, made massage, acupuncture, moxa cautery and bone-setting possible as occupations while at the same time making all other traditional therapies impossible as occupations. The law states:

> "All practices, other than those listed above,
>
> are quasi-medical professions."

In this way, massage, acupuncture, moxa cautery and bone-setting became institutionally approved, whereas all other traditional therapies, including Reiki, became disapproved. This marked a significant change in the field of therapies, as based on the prewar system they had been approved as occupations once registered with the local police office. Later, in 1960, more changes were made in relation to the 'freedom to choose occupation' section of the constitution. The Supreme Court stated that only quasi-medical practices that were harmful to human health would remain illegal. Thus, since then, many therapies, now called 'alternative therapies' have been practiced in a grey area. Even today in Japan, if I were to refer to myself as a therapist, it wouldn't be accepted by society who would see me as a 'would-be' therapist.

Other countries such as England, France and Germany did not face the same strict policies that GHQ executed in Japan. As a consequence, alternative therapies have been practiced there for a long time. There are organizations therapists can become affiliated with and people are more open and accepting of them.

When GHQ entered Japan, they designed the blueprint for the 'New Japan' and took steps to make it more scientifically advanced. Their aim was to change the mindset of the general public to have them believe that becoming modern and scientifically advanced was in everyone's best interests. One of the consequences of this is that alternative therapies like Reiki continue to be practiced in a legally and socially grey area.

## Propaganda spread by GHQ

GHQ spread propaganda systematically and thoroughly throughout Japanese society.

Some concerned the war. For example:

- *Japan is fully responsible for all war damage at home and abroad.*
- *Japanese must simply accept the consequences that a great number of their civilians were massacred in the firebombing of Tokyo and dropping of the atomic bombs.*

No criticism of the bombing by US was permitted. The data acquired after Hiroshima and Nagasaki was hidden and any photographs of the aftermath of the atomic bombs were taken out of circulation.

Other propaganda concerned prewar Japan:

- *Japan is a warmongering, old-fashioned country.*
- *Prewar Japan is akin to the dark ages.*

It is true the Japanese had believed they should die for their Emperor. Military power was huge at that time and had abused Shinto and the Emperor system, creating State Shinto which differed greatly from the original Shinto. However, GHQ propaganda attacked so much of traditional Japanese culture and the experience of the war itself was so traumatic that Japanese people began to harbor dark, negative impressions toward everything in prewar Japan. This blanket denial of Japanese culture and values represents the worst self-denial that has ever happened in Japanese history.

Today, Japanese people's awareness of the prewar period (including mine) remains biased and tainted. I was influenced by such propaganda in my youth, feeling at odds with Japanese elements and drawn to American culture. However, having lived in the US, learned Reiki and after examining historical facts, I now realize that our understanding and impressions of our own country have been largely based on implanted misunderstandings. Knowing the difference between Western Reiki and Traditional Japanese Reiki and seeing them both taught in Japan, it became shockingly clear to me that the Christian mindset is still prevalent in present-day Japan.

Ironically, non-Japanese people seem to have more interest in or feel an affinity with Shinto, the Emperors and their poems than Japanese. Jikiden Reiki, one of the traditional forms of Japanese Reiki, is now taught in more than 44 countries. This was an eye-opening discovery to me.

## The lost values of Japan

Countless Japanese cultural values have been lost or devalued as a result of the occupation. I have noticed their loss while studying prewar and wartime history, learning Jikiden Reiki and especially while teaching Jikiden Reiki and Japanese culture to non-Japanese. Below are some of those values.

Japanese tend to:
- treasure things that cannot be seen,
- value all physical matter (all physical things are seen as a gift from nature),
- value conformity and avoid conflict,
- place importance on an organization or group,
- leave self-assertions behind,
- emphasize professional expertise,
- act intuitively rather than logically,
- speak ambiguously rather than logically,
- control themselves,
- strive on their own,
- care about their ancestors,
- be proud of their own country,
- keep something precious private,

- maintain a relationship with a local shrine or temple,

- live in harmony with nature,

- respect the old,

- be humble,

- be polite,

- be quiet,

- master one area of expertise,

- seek fulfillment in their work,

- have a positive perception of humanity,

- have the sensitivity to care about other people,

- be capable of non-verbal communication,

- have the capacity to appreciate the present moment,

- sense seasons and nature,

- have awe before nature,

- be flexible enough to accept foreign cultures, and,

- understand the subtleties of life through the senses.

Some of these values may often be perceived negatively by present-day Japanese, as faults or as old-fashioned. We should realize however, that these perceptions were misunderstandings that have been implanted by postwar propaganda and the subsequent change in attitudes.

### The defeat of Japanese culture

Japan's defeat in the Pacific War resulted in the US occupation. In my view, more than scientific and technological defeat, this represents cultural and political defeat. In the run up to the war, Japan was not significantly inferior in military technology but was rather competitive with Western countries in areas such as naval and aircraft technology, for example, they had Zero fighter planes. However, they lacked the cultural and political ability to protect their own country. Unwise political decisions were made, exemplified by the reckless and violent acts of the Japanese Army in mainland China and by rashly waging war against the US, which was far superior in terms of power.

Much of the responsibility lies with the Japanese people themselves. They allowed the rise of such a military and political regime. Globally, Japan was a young country at the time, it hadn't really communicated with the outside world for 300 years. The country opened to global influence during the Meiji period, so in terms of being a global country, it was only 50 years old. Many people disagreed with the war from the beginning, but in order to maintain harmony among the people they did not speak out - the manifestation of a negative aspect of Japanese cultural values. Sadly, as a result of the war, Japan lost all the remarkable parts of its culture as well as the negative.

England, France, the US and Russia were all looking for an opportunity to win hegemony in Asia. If Japan had had a more solid foundation it may have redirected the helm of history and avoided the occupation. During a period when almost all other Asian countries had been colonized or were under the control of Western powers, Japan put up a great battle, its efforts something to be proud of. However, the country fell victim to atomic attack, lost the war and came under US occupation.

It was primarily a cultural defeat.

Japanese in the postwar period inevitably lost confidence, felt inferior and began to consider their culture as outdated, leading to uncritical acceptance of Western culture. Moreover, many Japanese felt they'd been deceived during the war and a victim mentality arose as they realized they had been recruited and exploited for the sake of nationalism when the war was originally supposed to protect themselves and their families.

Today, the Japanese know too little about themselves. Even recently, newspapers have fabricated stories emphasizing the shortcomings of Japanese culture during the war which were later proven to be untrue. So the people of Japan are partly responsible for this loss of cultural values. They do not understand their strengths and weaknesses well enough. Due to this lack of self-knowledge, Japanese people are unable to make up for their shortcomings - how can they when they don't even notice the loss of cultural values?

The question of whether they truly learned a lesson from the war is often asked. Unfortunately, because they do not fully understand the prewar period, wartime or the occupation, the answer is probably not. The education system in Japan is lacking in that it fails to teach these subjects, leaving it to individuals to have to research anything they would like to know.

I believe Japanese people feel the loss of their culture as something missing deep inside, but have no idea what it is.

## The loss of Reiki in Japan

After defeat in the war, Japanese Reiki therapy was facing fierce headwinds both institutionally as a result of GHQ policy and culturally as attitudes changed towards the non-scientific. Hands-on therapy, which is scientifically inexplicable came to be seen as wholly questionable in the public eye. As a result, the Usui Reiki Ryoho Gakkai, which used to have as many as 10,000 members in the prewar period has greatly declined, having approximately 300-400 members now (Toshitaka Mochizuki *Reiki: iyashino-te*).

As I explained in Chapter 6, there are surprisingly quite a few students among those who come to my Western Reiki school whose grandparents practiced traditional Japanese Reiki or hands-on therapy. However, of their parents, now in their 60s and 70s, almost none are practicing. This clearly demonstrates the magnitude of shift in values after the war.

In addition to the shift in values, the liberalization of religion in the postwar era is also relevant. Some religions had been oppressed by the government in the prewar period but afterwards were able to freely engage in missionary work, which is of course a wonderful thing. However, some religious groups began attempting to use hands-on healing on random people in the street. This led to misperceptions taking root in people's minds that hands-on therapy is suspicious or religious.

Interestingly, religious groups practicing hands-on therapy have expanded

119

since the war, whereas groups that had been practicing it as an alternative therapy have rapidly gone extinct in the postwar environment. This has not been helped by antisocial and subversive activities by cults such as *Aum Shinri-kyo* (オーム真理教), who orchestrated the sarin attack in Tokyo in 1995. Their activities have caused others, engaged in authentic spiritual activities, to be entirely misunderstood. Such misperceptions make it difficult for those Reiki practitioners who wish to promote Reiki as a home therapy.

**A glimpse of Japanese Reiki in the immediate postwar period**

Hoichi Wanami served as fifth president of the Gakkai. Wanami had a grandson, a professional violinist who is well-known to people familiar with classical music. His name is *Takayoshi Wanami* (和波孝禧 - born 1945) and he has a serious visual impairment. His mother, *Sonoko Wanami* (和波その子 - *Wanami*'s daughter-in-law), wrote a book about him. I purchased the book with a layperson's hope that she might have mentioned Japanese Reiki or her father-in-law, Hoichi Wanami. To my surprise, I found she actually had! This book was first published in 1976 (the 51st year of Showa). I was surprised that the word "Reiki" could be found in a book published that recently when it had become unknown to the general public.

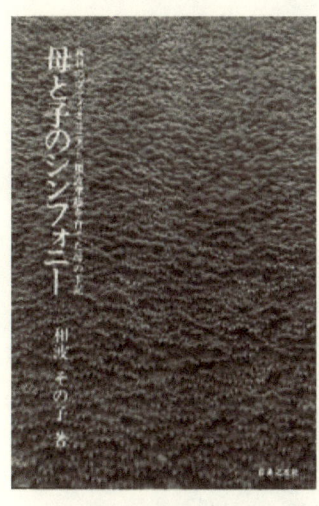

*Symphony of Mother and Child - Notebook of a Mother Who Raised Her Son, Takayoshi Wanami, a Blind Violinist by Sonoko Wanami* is available as a secondhand book at Amazon.co.jp. The 1976 and 1977 editions are the same in content. She also wrote a book entitled *Symphony of Life* but did not mention Reiki in that book.

I was deeply impressed by the book. It serves as a useful reference for Reiki and I would highly recommend it to Reiki practitioners and learners. Reiki actually appears in the early part of the book. I've chosen a few relevant passages to share:

"Dawn came quietly on the day of April 1st in the 20th year of Showa (1945). Although quite a few areas in central Tokyo seem to have been burnt down from daily air strikes, our neighborhood in an interior area of *Denenchofu*, having been attacked by a firebomb long ago, has remained quiet, if not for occasional roars in the sky (p.13).

"I heard my baby's first loud cry at 9:10am. The delivery was smooth....That night, the air strike was rather fierce with intensive bomb attacks reportedly hitting the area around Denenchofu station. Since my husband was already home, he hid my baby and me in the closet in the drawing room" (p.14).

People faced the constant fear of air strikes during that time, even in quiet suburbs like Denenchofu. The US repeatedly bombed civilians, women, children and the elderly indiscriminately in more than 200 cities. More than 700,000 civilians were killed (including more than 120,000 deaths in Hiroshima and 70,000 deaths in Nagasaki) while 15,000,000 people lost their homes. In this hostile environment, mothers were giving birth to and raising their children.

Such is life during a war.

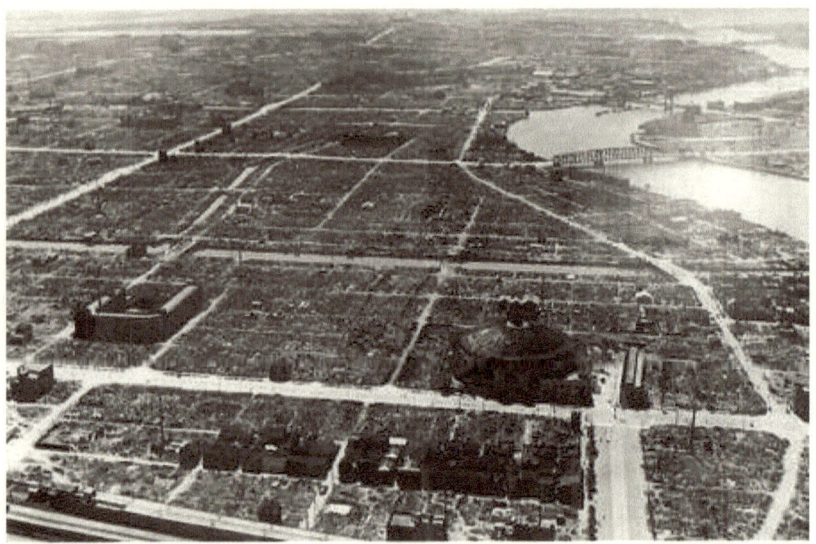

(East Tokyo after bombing on March 10, 1945, a picture by US airforce.)

"On August 15th, we were listening to the *Gyokuon* broadcast (the Imperial Rescript on Surrender) on the radio in the drawing room. My husband and I were sitting side by side and baby *Taka* was in my arms (p.20).

"While the news contained unsettling reports about such things as the occupying army, etc., our biggest concern was baby Taka's eye condition...following the advice '...you should take him to an appropriate hospital for a fundus (eye) examination', we visited the Naval Hospital in *Tsukiji*. Since we introduced our son as the grandson of Hoichi Wanami - a vice-admiral, or to be precise, a former vice-admiral - the doctor listened to us attentively, examining his eyes with various instruments in a dark room for some time" (p.21).

The Naval Medical School and Naval Hospital in Tsukiji have now been replaced by the National Cancer Center. This place is memorable for me as I have given Reiki treatments there in the past. Also, I went to an aromatherapy school in Denenchofu for a year, sometimes teaching as an instructor there. Because of these connections, I was able to relate to Sonoko's experience somewhat more directly.

"The fall in the 20th year (1945), the time following defeat in the war was a sad fall for my family as well....It was not until well into October that we decided to go for Reiki therapy as the sole available therapeutic option. The Reiki healer was an elderly person in *Harajuku*. I relied on that Reiki, or rather, it meant I could do something for him as a parent. How could I just sit back and watch my son growing up blind, simply feeding him milk every day? Ever since I heard that the father of my husband, Hoichi Wanami, did a number of experiments with Reiki, I presumed there was some mystical and logically inexplicable power in Reiki, and that it might work for baby Taka's eye condition, especially when the doctor could not even figure out its cause. The healer let him lie down and placed their fingers, through which Reiki flowed, on his forehead just above his eyes. The healer said, 'I can feel it',

> occasionally giving a groan and encouraged me by saying 'I can feel it so strongly that the optic nerve must be responding to it. It shall heal.' Baby Taka stayed calm in receiving the therapy" (p.28).

Sonoko was reconciled to raising her baby without his sight since the doctor had diagnosed him. Nonetheless, she continued to have him receive Reiki. The gender of, "an elderly person in Harajuku" in this section is unknown. He or she may have been related to the Gakkai, as it was initially headquartered in Harajuku. By saying, "It shall heal", he or she may have been perceiving byosen (病腺 the energetic sensation perceived in pathological areas); however, I personally wonder whether it was appropriate to assure full healing so optimistically.

Later, Sonoko also visited Dr. *Nishi*, the founder of *The Nishi System of Health Engineering* (see Chapter 12 for more detail), and started receiving guidance and incorporating remedies such as dietetics, including raw vegetables and raw unpolished rice, hot and cold baths etc. into everyday life.

> "I commuted to Harajuku for Reiki therapy every three days, carrying a lunch box for baby Taka which contained firm rice pudding simmered in milk....every now and then, on the path along the railroad toward Harajuku at dusk, I would often be overwhelmed with sorrow at the sight of the sunset over the barracks because it reminded me of *Toshiko* who had taken a path to *Yomi* (黄泉 the realm of the dead) earlier"(p.45).

Sonoko had lost her first daughter, Toshiko, who died of dysentery while in an evacuation area. She probably did not really believe that Reiki would heal her son's eyes, nevertheless, her wish for his healing as a mother would have driven her to commute to Harajuku so frequently for Reiki. Perhaps she wished that he would at least stay as healthy as possible. We can observe her wishes here though we have no specific details about his Reiki treatments throughout this period.

"Starting around March 25th (in the 21st year of Showa; 1946) the news began reporting the arrival of a repatriation train from Hainan Island. My mother, expecting our father's return, wanted to meet him and so I accompanied her to *Shinagawa* station. She wore *Mompe* (women's work pants).... and in this way, we commuted to Shinagawa station for three days in a row. On the afternoon of the 29th, when our mother stayed home as she was tired that day, we heard the doorbell ring and answered the door. It was our father..." (p. 45).

While Hoichi Wanami had joined a military reserve force in 1936, he seemed to have gone to the front by the end of the war according to this description. As Sonoko's biological father had been killed in battle in Rabaul in January 1945, the phrase 'our father', as used here, refers to her father-in-law Hoichi Wanami.

"He (Taka) played well, sang well, and grew well to greet the 22nd year (of Showa; 1947). I stopped commuting to Harajuku because his grandpa, a teacher of Reiki therapy, was there, who gave him a Reiki treatment from time to time..."(p. 50).

This implies that she had been commuting to Harajuku for Reiki for nearly two years. After Hoichi Wanami came back home, he had been performing the therapy. Quite surprisingly, no one else in this family other than Wanami was able to use Reiki.

Sonoko Wanami's book really brought my attention to something important. I am a Reiki teacher and as such, must pay attention to technique, methodology and the knowledge and information about Reiki. However, as crucial as all this is, the most fundamental thing for any practitioner to consider is the client. I realize that we must acknowledge that this is a human being who is sick or has a sick child, just like Sonoko Wanami. Without placing this in the centre of our awareness, the therapy would become a mere formality. With this in mind, I hope that when you perform Reiki for your family and for others, you focus on and feel their existence as a fellow human being.

Sonoko Wanami's second book entitled, *Symphony of Life* (1998), was written about her son, Takayoshi's adolescence. In it, she also describes the illness her husband (Hoichi Wanami's son) was fighting. However, she mentions nothing about Reiki in this book. Unfortunately, it is not clear how Reiki was used or how often it was utilized in the Wanami family. Sonoko's husband passed away in 1977, only two years after his father, Hoichi Wanami. It would be a pity if Reiki was lost in the family after that, however, if one of the family had continued with it, it would still remain hidden in the veil of secrecy covering the Gakkai.

## The mission of the Japanese

I think as Japanese people, we now have two obligations:

(1)  To heal the self-denial and loss of self-confidence that came from defeat in the war.

(2)  To reclaim the values of the original Japanese culture.

To my surprise, during my time overseas, I observed that a great number of non-Japanese are genuinely interested in the Japanese traditional culture of 'do' (道 'path' to something or 'way' of something). Examples of this culture are Judo (柔道 flexibility), Kendo (剣道 swordsmanship), Kyudo (弓道 archery), Sado (茶道 tea), Kado (華道 flower), Shodo (書道 calligraphy), and Koudo (香道 incense), as well as Bushido (武士道 samurai) and Shinto (神道 God). I realized how little Japanese people know and understand about their own culture. Of course, this is partly because Japanese culture has not been properly taught in schools since the war, but more significantly it is due to a lack of interest and independent study. Japanese should start studying themselves and their culture. Nowadays, many books, free from the influence of the postwar GHQ propaganda, are available. Using such books, simple study would easily reveal significant historical facts.

Japan tormented many neighboring countries and peoples during the Sino-Japanese War and the Pacific War. This is an undeniable fact which should be deeply reflected upon and learned from for the future. It does not

127

mean, however, that everything in the prewar period is to be rejected. Reflection and recognition need to be conducted in a fair manner.

Japan has a tremendous history extending over two thousand years. It carries a profound and rich culture that emerged from within that history and should be treasured. Japanese culture is so attractive and universal that an increasing number of non-Japanese show a keen interest in it. Needless to say, Reiki is one of those Japanese treasures.

# Chapter 9   The spread of Reiki to the West

Western Reiki is based on Japanese Reiki but was developed by Westerners as it spread throughout the world. It is now practiced by more than six million people. Let's have a look at how this development happened.

**Hawayo Takata - Reiki's first trip abroad**

Chujiro Hayashi and Hawayo Takata are responsible for the initial movement of Reiki outside Japan. Hayashi retired from the Navy in 1925 and (probably around 1929 when his name disappeared from the Gakkai member list) he started his own Reiki clinic in Shinano-machi, Tokyo which attracted a variety of clients. One of those clients was Hawayo Takata, a second generation Japanese American born and brought up in Hawaii (it is supposed the *yo* in *Hawayo* means a girl, and along with the first part - *Hawa*, it means girl born in Hawaii).

Takata developed serious health problems in her thirties. She travelled to Japan to have an operation, leaving her nine-year old daughter in the care of her Japanese relatives. It was October 1935 when she arrived in Yokohama with her daughter and, according to Helen Haberly's account of Hawayo Takata in her book, *Hawayo Takata's Story*, she was ready to undergo an operation when she heard an internal voice telling her it was not necessary. She chose not to go ahead with the operation, even though it must have felt awkward to the medical staff present, and decided to pursue other options. Takata's doctor's younger sister had been saved by using Reiki and she happily introduced Takata to Chujiro Hayashi. Fortunately, she made a complete recovery after receiving Reiki treatments for a few months at Hayashi's clinic. During this time she kept in contact with her doctor and went for regular checks to see how she was progressing. I will talk about her health issues more later.

Having made such a recovery, it was only natural that Takata become eager to learn Reiki so that she could use it herself on her return to Hawaii. People around her warned her that it would not be easy to learn and fully comprehend the nuances of the seminar contents given she was not a native Japanese immersed in the culture. However, she asked her doctor to write Hayashi a testimonial on her behalf (which would be a common thing to do in Japan under such circumstances) and as a result, Hayashi permitted her to join his classes.

After she learned Reiki, Takata worked at Hayashi's clinic for about half a year on an internship. It is guessed that she became a certified *shihan-kaku* (師範格 assistant teacher) prior to returning to Hawaii in June 1936.

On her return, Takata started to practice and teach the Reiki she had learned. More than 50 people in Hawaii joined Hayashi's institute and in July 1937 she visited Japan again, asking Hayashi to come and teach in Hawaii. He and his daughter *Kiyoe* (清枝) arrived in October of the same year, staying until February 1938. During this time he gave 14 seminars and welcomed 350 people as members of his institute. A photo exists of one of the seminars he held there, taken in Honolulu when Hayashi gave his final seminar on 19th February. This photo appeared in the Hawaii Hochi newspaper on March 4th 1938.

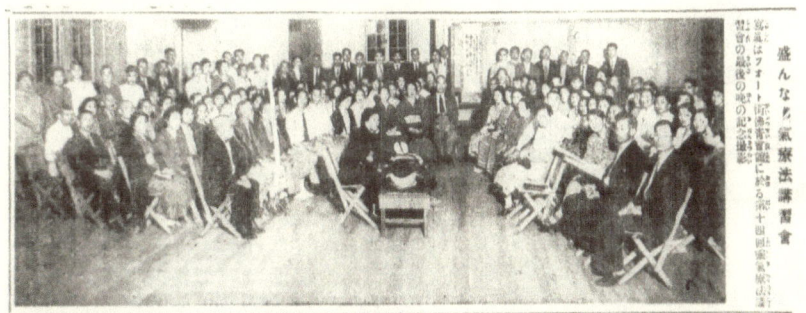

(Please note these are not participants of a single seminar but Hayashi's existing students gathered for commemoration.)

The information about Hayashi's trip to Hawaii comes from a farewell speech he made that was transcribed in the Hawaii Hochi newspaper on February 22nd 1938. The significance of this article lies in the fact that it is probably more accurate than other articles available because it was a speech he made as opposed to an article written by a journalist and his or her editor. (Thanks to Justin Stein of the University of Toronto and Hirano Naoko who found these important articles. Interested readers can visit his Web site at http://www.thescienceofsoul.wordpress.com)

I did a complete survey of the Hawaii Hochi newspaper articles and advertisements from September 1937 to June 1938 and was interested to find that 71 were related to Reiki. The detailed report can be seen at http://jikiden-reiki-nishina.com/hawaii/.

Takata's shihan (師範 teacher) certificate was issued in English by Hayashi on February 21st 1938, right before he returned to Japan. A photo of the certificate can be seen on page 301 of Frank Arjava Petter's book, *The Spirit of Reiki* (ISBN: 0914955675). The certificate states that she is certified as, *A master of the Usui Reiki system of drugless healing*, which was the origin of the title, Reiki Master, given to Reiki teachers in the west.

It was only three years after Hayashi's visit that the Pacific War erupted due to the Japanese attack on Pearl Harbor. Influential Japanese Americans in Hawaii were seen as enemies and put in concentration camps. These included corporate executives, teachers, Buddhist and Shinto monks, newspaper editors, fishermen, and anyone who seemed to be pro - Japanese or a potential threat to the US. Somehow, Hawayo Takata evaded this fate. Any group gathering with more than 10 Japanese was forbidden and use of Japanese language in public venues was banned. We cannot find any records of Takata's Reiki activities during the war and once it was over she didn't seem to be engaged in any public activities such as lectures or teaching, though there are a few records of her giving usual Reiki treatments in the 1950s and 60s.

During the 1970s Takata was urged to start training successors. She was in her mid-70s and given her cardiac condition realized she may not live very much longer. The total number of teachers she trained before she passed away in 1980, at the age of 80, was 22.

After her passing, the 22 teacher students founded various organizations and started progressively propagating Reiki. Around this time, the New Age movement in the West was growing. Spiritual books were being published regularly, New Age seminars were gaining popularity and new healing modalities were booming. These were great circumstances for Reiki to spread rapidly among people interested in this movement.

Through Hayashi, Hawayo Takata had brought Reiki to Western countries. The wave took hold and it quickly spread throughout the world.

## Takata's health problems

The information we have about Takata's health issues comes from books written by her students that give accounts of the stories she told them about her life.

---

Helen J. Haberl *Hawayo Takata's Story* ISBN 0944135064

[In Hawaii] From 1930 to 1935 she had little rest and finally suffered a nervous breakdown from overwork. In addition, she had sever physical problems - a painful abdominal condition which required surgery and respiratory problems which prevented the use of anesthetic. .................. She was not yet thirty-five years old, but she felt sixty, for she was unable to walk upright because of the pain in her abdomen. At times, she had great difficulty breathing. (page 17)

[At a hospital in *Akasaka*, Tokyo] It (her resting at the hospital) was three

---

weeks before he (her doctor) called her in for a thorough examination, and he confirmed she had a tumor, gallstones, and appendicitis, these being the cause of her abdominal pain. (page 19)

[At Hayashi's clinic] As their hands lightly touched her, they would comment on what they were sensing: "Oh, yes, your gall bladder is not too good; you must have a lot of pain here," and "There is a lump here; it could be a tumor," and so on. When they made such observations she could feel the heat from their hands, but she did not understand how they knew these things and wondered if the hospital had called them. (page 21)

Fran Brown *Living Reiki: Takata's Teachings* ISBN 0940795108

[In Hawaii] She had little rest, pushing herself to hide her grief, to the point where she had a nervous breakdown. She also had a painful abdominal condition, a uterine tumor which required surgery, and emphysema from asthma which prevented the use of an anesthetic. ........ [Takata said,] "I am not yet thirty-five years old, yet I feel like I'm sixty. I cannot walk upright because of the pain in my stomach. Often I cannot even breathe." (page 19)

[At *Maeda* hospital in *Akasaka*] Dr. *Maeda* took one look at her and promptly told her that she needed rest and comfort. ....... In three weeks, she was given a thorough examination along with x-rays and told, "You have a tumor, gall-stones and appendicitis. That's why your stomach aches all the time." (page 24)

> [At Hayashi's clinic] The gentleman who worked on her head told her that her eyes were taking a lot of energy. They needed to be revitalized. The other gentleman was treating her stomach from the right side of her body and said, "I feel you have lots of pain the area of the gall bladder." A little lower he said, "You have a lump... could be a tumor, and I'm feeling a lot of bad vibrations around your appendix." HOW COULD THEY TELL THAT? There was no time for the hospital to send around a diagnosis. (page 25)

These two books cover common ground so similarly that they presumably quite accurately recount what Takata had told her students. Unlike the tale of Usui's life that she had devised, these should be basically authentic as they are about her own life. We can therefore clearly confirm that the Reiki therapists perceived the problematic areas on her body through the sensations they felt in their hands. If you practice Japanese Reiki using the Byosen or Hibiki technique using your hands to make such conclusions is an ordinary and necessary part of treatment. As I describe in Chapter 11 Takata unfortunately stopped teaching this important technique to her students despite her experience as a patient. It is very odd that American Reiki practitioners did not take this information more seriously, it leaves me wondering why Takata's students did not question her in this regard.

**Takata after the war**

Very little information exists about how Takata practiced Reiki after the war. What we have can be found in written documents such as Fran Brown's book, *Living Reiki - Takata's Teaching* and John & Lourdes Gray's

*Hand to Hand* (ISBN 1401049605). John Gray, as the third teacher of 22 taught by Takata, learned and worked on Reiki with her for a relatively long time. A third book with information about Takata is *The Reiki Sourcebook* (ISBN 1846941814) published by Bronwen & Frans Stiene. This book is a collection of stories people have told and information taken from other books. In my opinion it does not appear to present objective references on the course of events and developments regarding Reiki at that time so we cannot be sure of the accuracy of the information.

Travel records show that Takata visited Japan in 1954, 1955 and again in 1957. *The Reiki Sourcebook* suggests that she travelled to Japan around 1950 and visited Hayashi's Reiki center but found it closed. Information from Helen Haberly's book and from Tadao Yamaguchi in Japan also indicates that Takata came to Japan and met Chie Hayashi, the wife of Chujiro Hayashi, so we can assume this information must have been true.

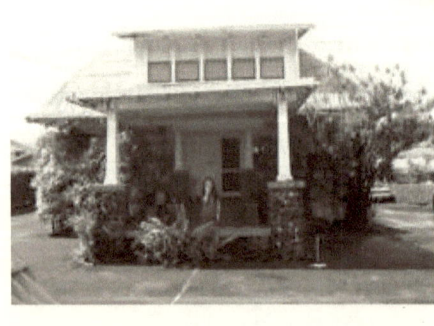

After the war, Hawayo Takata practiced Reiki in Hilo, a town on the East side of Hawaii island, which sits at roughly the same latitude as the well-known town of Kona on the West coast. The house in which Takata used to practice Reiki can still be found near Kilauea Street. Unlike Kona, Hilo receives a great deal of rain throughout the year and is therefore not a popular tourist destination. It is however, home to an office of the Japanese

National Astronomical Observatory and a base for the Subaru telescope on Mauna Kea. I used to be a member of the observatory and visited Hilo several times before coming into contact with Reiki and learning that Takata's house had been there.

Today, the house has a new owner and interestingly, is still used as the location for a therapy business, though not Reiki. The current owner discovered this wooden sign in the basement of the house. It belonged to Hawayo Takata and advertises her treatments. The house owner now displays the board realizing how precious it is.

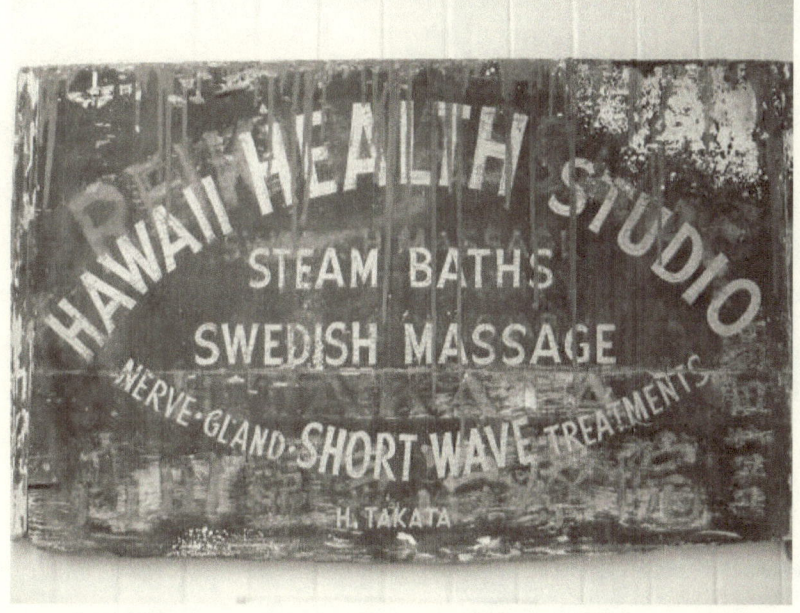

People who practice Reiki will probably be moved to tears to see this historic signboard. While it has been repainted at least once, you can make out what was written underneath through the paint. I used image processing to restore the original lettering as you can see in the second picture. It reads:

REIKI MASSAGE

SWEDISH MASSAGE

H. TAKATA

髙田靈氣治療院

(Takata Reiki clinic)

髙田ハワヨ

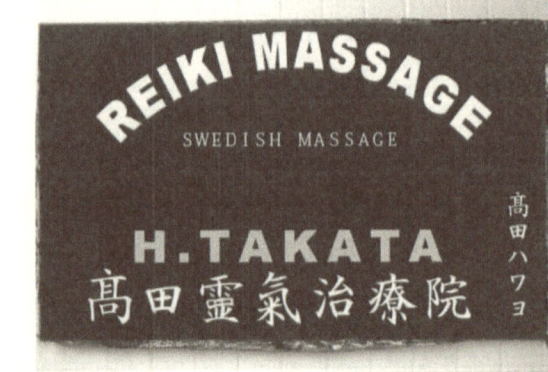

(Takata, Hawayo - written vertically on the right side)

According to documents found in this house, Takata purchased the property in 1939 and lived there until the 1950s when she moved to Honolulu. We can only guess at how Takata gave Reiki treatments in those days. According to the current house owner, it seems that she hired another therapist who practiced Hawaiian lomi lomi massage on the first floor while she practiced Reiki on the second floor of the house.

When the signboard was repainted the word Reiki and the kanji characters were removed. This seems significant and my guess is that the old lettering was used between 1939 and 1941 but after the Japanese attack on Pearl Harbor it was necessary to change it to avoid drawing attention to herself. It could have been done for other business reasons but the war must have had an influence. The new lettering remained there until the 1950s when she left the area.

*The photos of Takata's former house and the signboard were taken by Shoko Okazaki, a Reiki therapist living in Kona. Thank you, Shoko for your contribution.*

It is not known exactly what Reiki activities Takata was involved in after she left Hilo. We do know she was giving Reiki treatments in Honolulu. John Gray heard that Takata had become patronized by Doris Duke, the daughter of a millionaire, and had given her Reiki on a daily basis as her private therapist, attending her even when she traveled around the world. Official travel records show she did travel with Doris Duke to Guam in 1957 so this may well be accurate.

Takata resumed her teaching in the 1970s, first teaching Reiki only to Japanese Americans. She might have avoided teaching non-Japanese Americans for fear of facing the cultural differences, however, in 1973 she did teach some non-Japanese Americans for the first time. She began in Washington State, then gradually expanded the areas she traveled to teach both in the US and Hawaii. Eventually, having developed a heart problem and knowing she may well have to stop soon, she trained three Reiki teachers (one was John Gray) and wrote letters to those involved in Reiki confirming that those three teachers were to be her successors. Later however, she trained an additional 19 teachers from Hawaii, the US and Canada before passing away in 1980 at the age of 80.

## Takata - teaching Reiki

When Hawayo Takata taught her 22 student teachers, some techniques she had learned from Hayashi were either omitted or not taught thoroughly, while others she had not learned from him were added.

*The following techniques were NOT passed down⋯*


· *Byosen and shirushi for Byosen*

Byosen (病腺) means *disease gland or disease origin.*

This can be perceived by the practitioner as sensations of heat, tingling, itching, throbbing or pain in his or her hands. According to research by Robert Fueston, Takata taught Byosen to her students to some degree. In his book, *The History and System of Usui Shiki Reiki Ryoho* (ISBN 0997026804), he indicates that she told her students that during the treatment they should trust their hands, and listen to the vibration or reaction. She did not use the word Byosen and it appears she did not teach Byosen in a systematic way because her master students did not teach it and they did not recognize its importance. Instead, she devised standard hand positions as guidance. John and Lourdes Gray didn't refer to Byosen at all in their book, *Hand to Hand*. John placed high value on Takata's introduction of the standard hand positions which is a clear indication that he knew nothing or very little about Byosen.

The shirushi (印 - shirushi corresponds to a symbol in Western Reiki) for Byosen was not passed down by Takata either.

The word Byosen is a term used in Japanese Reiki. Hiroshi Doi, founder of Gendai Reiki (現代レイキ), substituted this with *hibiki* (響) meaning tremor in the late 1980s because Byosen sounds like something quasi-medical to post-war Japanese people.

## • Ketsueki Kokan Ho - a blood circulation method

Grays' book says that Takata practiced Ketsueki Kokan Ho (血液交換法), which is a blood circulation method, on her own clients. She called this method 'Reiki Finish'. She must have taught this method in Hawaii before the war as at the time she was teaching the same things Hayashi taught students when he visited Hawaii. In the US however, this massage-like technique cannot be performed openly without a proper massage license. Because of this restriction, John Gray did not teach this technique to his students. He substituted it with a procedure designed to produce similar effects, one that is not found in today's Western Reiki teachings anymore. The American International Reiki Association, one of the associations established by Takata's master students, dropped 'Reiki Finish' from their teaching before 1983.

## • Reiji-ho

Takata learned *Reiji-ho* (霊示法 miraculous finding method) from Hayashi in 1936 but the technique died out in Western Reiki. Reiji-ho is a technique to intuitively find compromised parts of the body. It is taught in Usui Reiki Ryoho Gakkai. Takata mentioned in her 1936 journal, *Mr. Hayashi has granted to bestow on me... Leiji-ho - the utmost secret in the energy science* (please note that native Japanese do not differentiate between the pronunciation of R and L). Takata seems to have taught this technique only to her students with intuitive ability. After the first generation of Takata's lineage, such intuitive techniques died out. Generally speaking, the intuitive techniques were not passed down in the Western

Reiki system.

### · *Ken-yoku - dry bathing*

I assume that Takata had not learned *Ken-yoku* (乾浴 dry bathing) from Hayashi. There is no record of Hayashi teaching Ken-yoku in Jikiden Reiki, while Gakkai people see this technique as important.

### · *Gokai - the five principles*

The English translation of the Gokai was passed down among Takata's students. However, when it was translated into English it lost its kotodama or word spirit which is held in the original Japanese and considered of great importance. In addition, the concepts of *Gyo* (業) and *hageme* (励め) are not present in Western culture. *Gyo wo hageme* (業を励め) is different from *work hard* or *work diligently*. Unfortunately, this was unavoidable and often happens in a process of translation.

### *The following techniques were ADDED or changed...*

### · *Standard hand positions*

As I mentioned in the section on Byosen above, Takata developed standard hand positions so a treatment is given on designated parts of the body in a particular order. Her teacher student, John Gray, did read Hayashi's treatment guide as a copy had been left in Hawaii, but he got the mistaken impression that it was confusing. Hayashi's guide indicates which areas of the body are treated for various conditions. Often it suggests several positions for a single symptom, and similar combinations of positions for

142

widely different symptoms. However, John Gray's confusion was simply an unfortunate misunderstanding. If a practitioner hasn't studied Byosen, he or she can easily assume Hayashi's guide is directing them to give Reiki to all the body parts in a listed order. The areas indicated are not a treatment directive though, they are the areas a practitioner is most likely to perceive Byosen sensations on his or her hands. Therefore, it is simply a handy guide suggesting which areas to pay attention to when looking for Byosen. Jikiden Reiki practitioners know that Hayashi never suggested his students give Reiki on all the designated parts in order.

I am truly puzzled as to why Takata stopped teaching Byosen or didn't teach it thoroughly and focused only on standard hand positions. She must have been well-informed about Byosen given that she worked as an intern at Hayashi's clinic in Tokyo for around six months. John Gray, having misunderstood the process and the guide, over-valued the fact that Takata created standard hand positions. Nevertheless, this concrete method of easy-to-follow hand positions has been appreciated greatly by Western practitioners. As I discuss in Chapter 11, Americans seem to prefer more clear-cut and standardized approaches than Japanese.

Takata's standard hand positions consist of seven basic positions - four on the abdominal area and three on the head. Extra positions can be added if necessary depending on the client's needs. John Gray developed his own version of the hand positions based on these as he explains in his book. However, today, the standard hand positions taught in Western Reiki systems are different from either of the those above. They were established by Reiki practitioners succeeding Takata and her students.

### • *Aura and chakras*

Takata did not teach the concepts of auras or chakras. Her students, those such as John Gray and later generations, introduced these ideas from modalities such as Indian Ayurveda and various New Age techniques. Similarly, the Western lineage of Reiki began to embrace and legitimize the concepts of cleansing objects and purifying places.

### • *Reiki shower*

There is some information about a ritual that may be similar to the idea of Reiki shower in the Gakkai, but I'm not sure if they are the same. Hayashi did not teach anything similar. However, Yoga teachers often use a similar technique. I will continue to investigate this.

### • *Attunements*

Takata's students say that they remember her attunements being done differently each time. She followed her hunch at the time and changed it accordingly. It is unclear when today's Western Reiki attunements were established.

### • *Symbols and mantras*

The symbols and mantras known in the Western Reiki systems today do stem from Hayashi's teaching, however, it is not known when or how they evolved and were modified from the original shirushi and jumon of Japanese Reiki. It is also not known if this modification was made by

Takata herself or her students. Somewhere along the way, a wide variety of changes and misunderstandings were brought into all elements of the practice of symbols and mantras.

## Mantras

It is important to know that the mantras were added by Western people in the Reiki system. Originally, the shirushi were always used without any chanting. Only the jumon is used in conjunction with a chant in Japanese Reiki.

## Shirushi for Byosen

Because the Byosen technique was not taught in the Western system of Reiki the shirushi for Byosen was not taught either. It is important not to make the mistake of thinking this shirushi is CKR, which came from an entirely different shirushi.

## The first symbol

CKR: Takata taught this in her level 2 class as a command meaning, *All scattered energy, gather immediately*. A similar form is used in Japanese Reiki but for different purposes and on different occasions. Therefore, using CKR like this is something Takata developed incorrectly in terms of Japanese Reiki. The mantra connected to CKR in Western Reiki, *choku rei*, is actually an incorrect reading of the original kanji characters 直霊. These characters can be read correctly if one has knowledge of Shinto. It is very puzzling that Takata taught it incorrectly.

*The second symbol*

SHK: A similar-shaped figure is used for *seiheki chiryo* (mind-habit treatment) in Japanese and Western Reiki. However, the concepts behind them and the techniques used are different. Takata taught SHK as a 'deprogramming' technique and told students to make a positive suggestion concerning the habit, which is very different from in the Japanese Reiki. The important kotodama (word spirit) students learn for seiheki chiryo was lost here.

It is important to know that what has become a mantra in the West, the word seiheki, means *bad habit* in Japanese. Imagine chanting, "bad habit, bad habit, bad habit" when you treat someone. It sounds quite funny to Japanese people.

*The third symbol*

HSZSN: Something very similar is used for distant treatments in Japanese Reiki, too. There is little alteration here but readers should know that many distorted versions of HSZSN have been created in the Western Reiki system and some teachers have even posted YouTube videos that show it written in the incorrect order while stating it is the correct order.

*The Master symbol*

DKM: This is entirely the creation of Western culture. DKM has never existed in Japanese Reiki. The basic concept of DKM is inconsistent with Japanese Reiki. This symbol is the key that differentiates Western Reiki and Japanese Reiki. If a system teaches or uses DKM, it must come from the Western tradition, but we do not know for sure who introduced it. I give a thorough explanation of this in Chapter 11.

I understand that some of the changes in these symbols and mantras were introduced with good intention, but they reflect the Western way of thinking and undermine the possibility of understanding Japanese Reiki.

## Takata - difficult decisions

Despite learning Reiki directly from Hayashi, when Takata came to pass it on it was with a different flavor. She made the necessary choices around which techniques to adapt or leave in order to ensure Reiki would spread in the US. Her students in turn broke new ground by developing their own styles of Reiki with a distinctly Western taste.

It seems Takata didn't teach Byosen thoroughly which is the most important technique used for medical treatment in Japanese Reiki. This is surprising given that it was used to save her from the life-threatening conditions she faced, and that during her six months as a live-in student at Hayashi's clinic she must have encountered a great many cases where Reiki was used medically. According to Fran Brown's *Living Reiki: Takata's Teachings*, Takata told her students not to take notes or keep records of Reiki treatments because they could be seen as diagnosis, even if unintentional, which was a violation of law. She spoke to them about leaving this kind of diagnosis to medical professionals and seems to have been overly concerned about the issue. It is true that by law in both the US and Japan, one cannot diagnose or medically treat patients unless engaged in a medical profession, so it may be that she concluded that in order to propagate Reiki she would have to reduce the medical elements. If that was the case, it must have been a tough decision for her.

I would like readers to know that teaching Byosen to Western students, who have a different cultural background, is not difficult at all. For example, I have taught Jikiden Reiki to more than fifty Hungarian students and most of them could perceive Byosen during the seminars and learned how to utilize it well, probably even better than Japanese students.

Trainings and exercises for self-cultivation, plus emphasis on practice and experience are other elements that disappeared as Reiki transformed from Japanese to Western Reiki, where it was emphasized that Reiki does not require trainings or practices. To compensate for this, great importance has been placed on the power of symbols and mantras. Instead of working internally, they rely on the power of these to enhance their healing. This emphasis on symbols and mantras has brought its own set of problems which I discuss in Chapter 11.

The approach of lowering the hurdle has achieved the aim of spreading Reiki, but has not benefited highly motivated practitioners who may lose the impetus for self-cultivation. In today's fast-paced, over-stimulated world, we are all encouraged to want the quick, cheap and easy way in life and in Reiki. I call this, *McDonald-ized Reiki*.

Another reason Reiki spread so widely after Takata was the significant decrease in tuition fees for Reiki courses. It became affordable and available to anyone wanting to learn. In pre-war times, the cost of taking a traditional Japanese Reiki course and becoming shihan (teacher) was significantly higher.

Spiritual healing, in which the physical condition of a client is not a main concern was a new element introduced into Western Reiki, which was welcomed by those who are looking for a more peaceful and compassionate mind. The result of this is that many Western Reiki practitioners do not use Reiki when they become sick. In Japanese Reiki mind and body are closely related.

Takata's courageous decisions allowed Reiki to pass from her, as a single teacher, to millions of people. Without all the changes it underwent, it would have been wholly impossible for the countless Reiki practitioners in the world today to be so active. Because of this, I think we must greatly appreciate the McDonald-ized Reiki that serves a dollar coffee or hamburger and gives temporary peace of mind.

And we must look forward to a more nutritional diet that helps us grow and sustains us.

### The spread across the globe
Today Reiki is practiced all over the world. So much so, it is easier to list the countries where Reiki is not practiced than those that have embraced it.

African countries with few caucasians, Arabian countries that disassociate with the West and China, where Qi-going is commonly practiced have little or no Reiki. Aside from these regions, Reiki has expanded across the globe. It has even been brought into Thailand and Bali, regarded wholly as Buddhist countries, by the Caucasians and Japanese residing there. In resorts such as Hawaii Reiki has been commonly adopted as a treatment menu in spas. In the West, a number of people have found its efficacy as alternative medicine, encouraging it to be practiced in hospitals and medical facilities. The number of Reiki lovers all over the world continues to grow.

## Takata - the contrast with Usui Reiki Ryoho Gakkai

Takata and the Gakkai show a remarkable contrast in their approaches to Reiki. Takata promoted Reiki by modifying it for Western taste while the Gakkai stuck stubbornly to tradition. Let's look at the differences between these two approaches.

### Takata's approach

Hawayo Takata taught a variety of fictitious stories in her Reiki classes including false accounts of Usui being a Christian priest, president of Doshisha University (a Christian school) and that he studied in Chicago University. Some of these stories, along with others she told are still published today in Western Reiki books. Though false, Takata's stories had a purpose. They must have helped Reiki to be accepted by Hawaiian residents whose fellow countrymen and women were killed by the Japanese attack on Pearl Harbor.

In addition, as I have mentioned, Takata gave up the techniques of importance for treating diseases, changing Reiki from a physical remedy to a spiritual healing modality. She purposefully stepped away from maintaining tradition in service to the spread of Reiki. Having undergone Takata's modifications, Reiki became recognized and energized by the New Age and Spiritual Movements, circulating the world with relative ease.

In my opinion, Takata gave people what they wanted at the time.

## The Gakkai's approach

While Western Reiki circumnavigated the globe, its Japanese counterpart concealed the practice after the war and continues to do so today.

By refusing to change or to keep abreast of the times, the Gakkai failed to promote Reiki to the general public which is a great loss for Reiki, a precious asset to humanity.

## A Japanese perspective

Nowadays, thanks to the efforts of motivated Reiki practitioners, people are getting access to the correct history and stories around Reiki. Despite some authors condemning Takata for passing down false information and altering the original Japanese Reiki, her decision to do this not only enabled people to access Reiki in the West, it also led us all to find the original Japanese Reiki. Even Jikiden Reiki would not have been taught by the Yamaguchis if Takata had not existed because their motivation to teach publicly was initiated when they discovered the existence of Western Reiki.

Takata was able to achieve what she did because she was a Japanese American rather than a native Japanese. If she had been born and brought up in Japan, she may well have been persistent in keeping the Japanese tradition and not had the courage to make all those changes for the Western palette.

The antipodal approaches of Takata and the Gakkai gave vastly contrasting experiences of Reiki to the communities in the West and Japan. I am certain that Takata made the right choice.

**The importance of women in Reiki**

Women have played impressive roles in the history of Reiki. During Usui's lifetime, there were already a great many women practitioners as can be seen in group photographs taken at the time. Such photographs can be found in The Hayashi Reiki Manual by Tadao Yamaguchi and Frank Arjava Petter as well as in Toshitaka Mochizuki's book, *Choo Kantan Iyashi no Te* (ISBN: 4812701430). *Choo Kantan Iyashi no Te* means *Very Easy Hand Healing*. This second book of Mochizuki's is not translated but carries a great deal of important information and includes some interesting photographs. Other group photos taken after Hayashi's Reiki classes show many female participants (these photos belong to the Jikiden Reiki Institute in Japan). Still today, Reiki is practiced overwhelmingly by women. In the Reiki classes I teach, eight out of ten students are women.

Women haven't just been practitioners of Reiki, in actuality, the path of Reiki from past to present has been paved primarily by women! Takata was the forerunner, without her Reiki would not have reached the West. Kimiko Koyama, sixth president of the Gakkai seems to have been very active too. If she hadn't introduced Hiroshi Doi to the Gakkai, some of the traditional Reiki information may not have been available today. She must have had a firm vision for the future. Last, but by no means least, Chiyoko Yamaguchi of Jikiden Reiki. Although the official activity was started by her son, Tadao Yamaguchi, Chiyoko was the one who practiced Reiki consistently throughout the time of war and onward. Without Chiyoko, we would never have come to know the true teachings of Hayashi as they were in his day.

You may remember that in Chapter 6 I introduced five women whose stories also contribute to our understanding of Reiki through time. Women seem to possess a stronger, more enduring life force than men when it comes time to put things forward. Men tend to have a somewhat simplistic, egoistic and society-oriented nature, thus they are generally good at setting goals and taking initiative. They may well proceed at full speed when getting recognition from society, but are not so good at making a steady effort in the face of little or no fame or status and therefore tend to stop if they can't obtain social status or recognition. Women, on the other hand, will work diligently, even without such social status or recognition and will slowly and surely persist.

In terms of Reiki, women have been using it to play a major role in taking care of their family members' health. Consequently, they have been the ones who tend to use Reiki on a daily basis. Women's devotion to family, along with their tenacity, has been a great driving force for the revival of Reiki today.

Throughout my teaching and practicing Reiki, I have been encouraged by women's deep love and strong will to keep their family healthy and I have been learning from them about how we need persistence to spread Reiki to more people.

# Chapter 10   The Return of Reiki to Japan

In the aftermath of the war, Reiki lost the public recognition it had previously enjoyed and the healing art died out until it was only practiced by a handful of people who had to be discreet in their use of it.

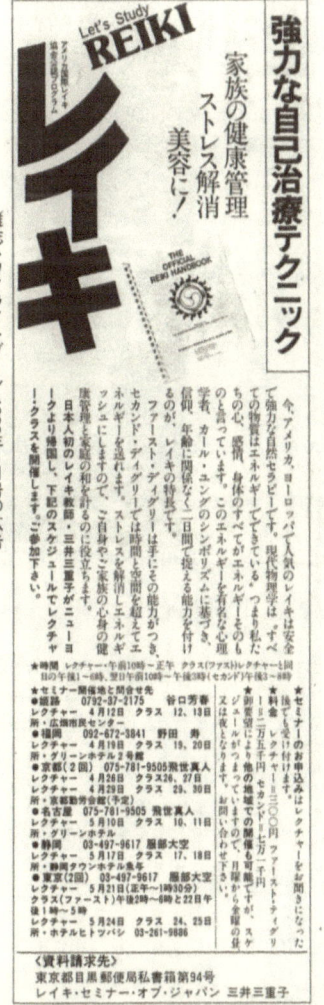

Much later, in the 1980s, it was re-imported as Westernized Reiki which came from the United States. As a result there was a difference in the way the word Reiki was written. Japanese Reiki is written as 靈氣 or 靈気 while this imported Western Reiki was phonetically written as レイキ, where レ is for Re, イ is for i, and キ is for ki. The three different ways of writing Reiki are pronounced the same.

It was Mieko Mitsui, a journalist living in New York who first brought Western Reiki into Japan. Mitsui was a teacher from the Radiance Technique, one of the Reiki organizations in the US. It was 1984 when she started teaching and giving attunements in Japan. On the left is an advertisement for one of Mitsui's workshops in 1986. Within the text it says, "Reiki is a safe, powerful, natural therapy popular in the US and Europe.... Mieko Mitsui, the first Japanese teacher of Reiki, comes back from New York and ...".

In 1987 Mitsui translated a book by Barbara Ray, founder of the Radiance Technique, into Japanese. In English the book was titled, The Reiki Factor (ISBN: 0933267061) while in Japanese it became *Reiki Ryoho* (Reiki Therapy). Though Mitsui was teaching in Japan, she was only qualified to teach up to the second degree (level 2) and therefore was not able to teach teachers. Hence, people still could not easily find a Reiki teacher in Japan.

The situation changed when Frank Arjava Petter started teaching in Hokkaido, a northern island of Japan. From 1993 he offered full courses in Western Reiki including the teacher's level. Japanese people began to establish their own Reiki schools on completing Petter's course. This gifted more and more people the chance to learn Western Reiki and was a catalyst for the spread of Western Reiki in Japan. Toshitaka Mochizuki, one of Petter's students started his own Western Reiki school with a man named Takahashi, who was also attuned by Petter. In 1995 Mochizuki published a Western Reiki book titled, *Iyashi no Te* (癒しの手 healing hands) which greatly contributed to the spread of Western Reiki in Japan. Reiki gradually started to gain more recognition among Japanese people as other leaders in the field followed this trend. It's only been around 25 years since Western Reiki was fully introduced into Japan, this is one of the reasons the general public here aren't so familiar with it yet.

In the 1980s and 90s people were practicing Western Reiki not knowing anything about Japanese Reiki. Only the things Takata spoke of were known, she had become something akin to a Reiki Bible in the Western Reiki community.

## Revival of the original Reiki

From the late 1990s, information on Japanese Reiki began to appear from several sources. Hiroshi Doi, who became a member of the Gakkai, published some traditional information in his book, *A Modern Reiki Method for Healing* (English edition ISBN: 1886785333) published in 1998. His information was somewhat limited though as he was not even shihan-kaku (assistant teacher) and was not allowed to reveal any technical details. He also mixed traditional information with Western Reiki because he had learned Western Reiki prior to joining the Gakkai. Despite these limitations many Western Reiki practitioners were enlightened by his book.

Frank Arjava Petter published *the Original Reiki Handbook of Dr Mikao Usui* (ISBN: 0914955578) in 1999, which was the translation of a small handbook edited by the Gakkai. The original Usui Reiki handbook had been passed down in the Gakkai but not known to the general public until Petter revealed it in his book. In fact, this was the first genuine Japanese Reiki literature to become public. The book disclosed some techniques of the traditional Usui Reiki system and its philosophy.

A definitive change occurred in 1999 when Chiyoko Yamaguchi (山口千代

子) and her son Tadao Yamaguchi (山口忠夫) started teaching Japanese Reiki under the name of *Jikiden Reiki* (直傳靈氣 Directly Taught Reiki). Chiyoko and her many relatives learned Reiki directly from Chujiro Hayashi in the 1930s and had been using Reiki since that time. By chance they discovered that Western Reiki was becoming popular in Japan and resolved to teach Japanese Reiki in order to give people access to the original Reiki. Western Reiki had awakened the sleeping Japanese Reiki! To clarify what and how Hayashi taught Reiki, Chiyoko and Tadao Yamaguchi visited their relatives to collect notes, photographs and their recollections. Their efforts brought about a complete recovery of Hayashi's teaching. Therefore, the contents of Jikiden Reiki are based not only on Chiyoko Yamaguchi's memory, but also the information kept by her relatives.

Jikiden Reiki allows anyone to learn Japanese Reiki, completely free from postwar Western influence. It is the first time since the war that Japanese Reiki has become fully available to the public. I attended my first Jikiden Reiki seminar in 2005.

Some information on Japanese Reiki is now publicly available through books such as *Light on the Origins of Reiki* by Tadao Yamaguchi and *The Hayashi Reiki Manual* by Frank Arjava Petter and Tadao Yamaguchi. Therefore, many Western Reiki practitioners nowadays, especially in Japan, know a little about Japanese Reiki, making the two Reiki groups closer. Many Western Reiki teachers in Japan more or less incorporate the information from these books into their curriculum.

Although the Gakkai still exists today, it is not possible for usual people to join without a reference from an existing member. As I have mentioned previously, Gakkai members are only allowed to practice Reiki on other members or their family and it is impossible to know what their activity is today. Reiki has become so popular in the world that they might find, 'coming out' even harder now.

## Frank Arjava Petter

Frank Arjava Petter introduced all levels of Western Reiki to Japan. Initially, he learned Reiki in the Reiki Alliance lineage, but later trained students independently of any schools. The majority of Western Reiki teachers in Japan can be traced back to Petter.

Petter patiently searched out and visited various places relevant to Reiki and met with a number of people that helped him dig up and clarify accurate information on Japanese Reiki. We owe him a great deal for revealing so much information on Japanese Reiki.

Petter has written a number of books on Reiki, one of which was *the Original Reiki Handbook of Dr Mikao Usui* I mentioned earlier. He also obtained a booklet written by Kimiko Koyama of the Gakkai and revealed the traditional techniques it contained in his books, *The Spirit of Reiki* and *This is Reiki* (ISBN: 0940985012). Another of his books, *The Hayashi Reiki Manual*, written with Tadao Yamaguchi of Jikiden Reiki, introduces precious information from Hayashi and some traditional Reiki techniques to the world.

Frank Arjava Petter has made such an enormous contribution to the revival of Reiki in Japan as well as the rest of the world. Nevertheless, he is not always recognized highly enough, especially in Japan. Perhaps this is because he did not belong to any particular organization, instead working independently. In addition, he did not publish his books in Japanese until 2015 which would be a contributing factor.

Petter's approach is quite contrary to that of Toshitaka Mochizuki who established his school of Western Reiki as a business. Mochizuki aggressively promotes his school through publications and advertisements to attract people to his workshops. Although this approach has greatly contributed to the spread of Western Reiki in Japan, I have a far closer affinity with Petter's independent approach.

In his book, *The Spirit of Reiki*, Petter indicated that he felt alienated in the Japanese community of Western Reiki since he is not Japanese. He wrote:

Even though I was the first person in Japan to openly teach all levels of Western Reiki, I still have not been accepted into the group of people who learned from me because I basically do not exist for them!
(page 141)

I would like to emphasize that his contributions deserve greater and wider recognition. I also think his other books should be translated into Japanese.

In 2000, Petter learned Jikiden Reiki directly from Chiyoko Yamaguchi. After that, he greatly reduced his teaching of Western Reiki and focused on the activities in Jikiden Reiki. It is very impressive that such a person who has mastered all the techniques in various versions of Western Reiki has finally been convinced by Japanese Reiki. Nowadays, he is recognized well among Jikiden Reiki people and has taken the post of vice-representative of the Jikiden Reiki Institute. Petter's enthusiasm for Reiki has finally been given the acceptance and recognition it deserves in Japan.

# Chapter 11    A Comprehensive Look at the Differences Between Japanese and Western Reiki

How different is Japanese Reiki from Western Reiki? And what exactly are those differences?

These would be natural questions asked by those who have learned Western Reiki. In this chapter, I would like to answer as fully as possible, which means taking into account not only the differences but the cultural backgrounds that produced them. To my knowledge there has, as yet, been no book that has studied differences in Reiki in terms of cultural background. Understanding the culture anything comes from gives a vital depth of understanding that cannot be found any other way.

In Chapter 9 I looked at how Takata was already teaching Reiki a little differently than she had learned from Hayashi. As Reiki has spread worldwide, it has continued to evolve and been further modified to become the Western Reiki we know today.

In this chapter I will not go into technical details which are to be taught in seminars and please be advised that the following comparison is based on my own view and understanding. You will see that despite the similarity of Japanese and Western Reiki, some elements are in fact very different. Some Western Reiki practitioners may feel uncomfortable since I am occasionally quite critical of some types of Western Reiki, however, I ask you to bear with me, I am simply looking at factual information and in no way 'attacking' Western Reiki. I have taught more than 2,000 Western Reiki students and understand the beneficial elements of Western Reiki too.

Before I begin, I'd like to define the meaning of *Western Reiki*. It is not easy to define because there are so many variations of Western Reiki. Depending on the type of Western Reiki a person has learned he or she may find they think Japanese Reiki is very different, or that it is somewhat similar to what they have learned.

In this book, Western Reiki is generally referring to Reiki taught by the Reiki Alliance and the Radiance Technique along with all Usui-shiki Reiki and Shiki Reiki. In Japan, Western Reiki refers to the Reiki taught at Vortex, a school run by Toshitaka Mochizuki. Gendai Reiki, established by Hiroshi Doi is also Western Reiki. Gendai Reiki did adopt a part of what Doi learned in Usui Reiki Ryoho Gakkai, but it is definitely a kind of Western Reiki. Doi is not shihan, or even shihan-kaku in the Gakkai and is not allowed to teach any of their techniques to non-Gakkai members. Later I will explain more about why Gendai Reiki is Western Reiki, which becomes obvious once you learn Jikiden Reiki.

*Usui-shiki* is an expression Ms. Takata started to use and is now commonly used in Western countries. In Western countries, especially in the US, people developed many different things they called Reiki, introducing various energies such as, love, the Universe, angels and a variety of gods sometimes imported from other cultures and ideologies such as yoga or shamanism. In principle, one can create infinite numbers of energies by introducing other energies into Reiki. Those who create these often call them *evolved Reiki*. This is a misunderstanding. Let me emphasize that ***Reiki is the energy that flows out unintentionally when one is in a natural state***. Reiki stands out from other types of healing because its energy has no intentions. There is therefore only one kind of Reiki energy. If other energies are mixed up in it, it is of course still an energy healing, useful for certain purposes, but it is certainly not Reiki any more. So, particularly in the US, the word Reiki has been skewed and come to mean *anything*. To avoid confusion, people have called the normal Reiki, Usui-shiki Reiki or Shiki Reiki for short. This situation only occurs in Western countries because these other 'evolved Reiki' systems are not popular in Japan. I do not deal with these in this book because they are not Reiki any more according to my definition.

Lastly, I'd like to clarify that the term, *traditional Reiki* in Western countries doesn't mean Japanese Reiki, it refers to Usui-shiki Reiki. Japanese people get very confused by this.

## The differences incorporating cultural perspectives

### The fundamental energy

The Reiki energy used in both Western Reiki and Japanese Reiki is essentially the same if we focus on the energy itself. Though I have learned both, I am not aware which energy I am using when I simply apply my hands.

Reiki flows out unintentionally when one is in a natural state, so of course, other animals also flow Reiki. Because it exists independent of human consciousness, intention, culture or religion, the energy itself cannot be characterized as anything - for example, it is not Oriental, Western, Arabic, traditional or modern.

However, once humans use the Reiki energy with particular techniques based on a certain consciousness, purpose, culture, worldview and/or religion, this universal energy can be used for a variety of purposes. This is how Western Reiki was able to evolve from Japanese Reiki using the same energy, and it is what makes Western Reiki and Japanese Reiki different.

I see problems among quite a number of Western Reiki practitioners. Some Western Reiki schools mistakenly tell students to use personal intention, imagination and/or deliberate breath. Such techniques introduce different energies into healing sessions, therefore, they are no longer pure Reiki. Most Western Reiki teachers and practitioners doing this are unaware of what energies they are dealing with.

In the following passages however, I assume the Reiki energy itself is the same in Western Reiki and Japanese Reiki.

*Dependence Vs self-reliance*

How one sees human beings and their relationship to all things is key here. The difference between typical Western Reiki and Japanese Reiki is represented in two contrasting basic concepts:

## Something given from outside Vs Something innate

In Western Reiki, one is able to use Reiki only after the ability has been given to them from outside, in the form of an attunement. It is not therefore, an innate ability but something given to them by others. There is also a strong tendency to depend on symbols and mantras which are given to them by others. Participants often pay fees for the attunements and symbols/mantras that are believed to transform a *normal* person into a *Reiki-able* person. This Reiki is therefore based on an understanding that one is entirely dependent upon others.

In Japanese Reiki, conversely, Reiki is an ability that everyone possesses innately. Master Usui clearly states in his public teaching:

> All living creatures, once their lives are given, commonly possess a mysterious healing ability as a heavenly blessing. This ability can be seen in grasses, trees, animals, fish and insects, and is best realized in humans because human beings are spiritual leaders.

Here, Reiki is self-reliance.

This difference in how one sees human beings determines how Western Reiki is different from Japanese Reiki in every corner. As I explain below most of their differences can be well understood from this point of view.

### *Religion*

I think Western Reiki is strongly influenced by Christianity, in which all humans are born with original sin. In this context we are all sinners in need of a salvation that can only come from outside us. One of the core objectives of this religion is therefore the saving of such powerless sinners.

Japanese culture and thinking is entirely different. Japanese Reiki is most likely highly influenced by Shinto, in which we are all branches of the great existence, with unbroken connections to it. Of course, while living in this secular world one may develop a vicious mind, but Shinto allows us to restart life afresh through a purification ceremony called, Misogi (禊ぎ). In addition, with a high level of discipline, one becomes capable of performing amazing things.

In Christianity or Buddhism, if one does wrong in this world, one would be thrown into hell. In some types of Christianity one can avoid hell by believing in Jesus and letting him 'save' them, but there is still no possibility of self-salvation or self-reliance. The choice is punishment or dependence. In Shinto, even if one commits a crime there would be no hell waiting. Instead, one's spirit simply goes back to the source upon death. No one is to be punished in Shinto.

In every aspect of Japanese Reiki, humans are an innately wonderful existence in this world. This is very different from Western Reiki where humans are seen as innately weak sinners.

### Mercy and affection
Something wonderful Christianity has brought to Western Reiki is the

concept of mercy and affection. In Japanese Reiki, in the Sei-heki chiryo or mind-habit therapy, the concept of mercy is present, but to a limited extent. Even when Shinto tells us everyone is innately strong, a weakened and depressed personality may feel they don't know what to do with the great difficulties he or she is facing. Western Reiki however, offers sympathy and healing to such a weakened person. Even when feeling deeply powerless, a person can easily use Western Reiki tools to feel secure, healed and even saved. It provides effectively for a person who has the earnest desire to be given something, to be treated gently, helped and saved.

## *Lineage*

Western Reiki bears a strong tendency towards relying on others and it is thought that people cannot use Reiki until the ability has been given by another through an attunement. In other words, the ability is transmitted from teacher to student. This gives rise to the idea that lineage is imperative - the closer to Master Usui, the better.

This idea of lineage is totally wrong!

I have given Western Reiki attunements to at least a couple of thousand people and I have felt Reiki coming out of many people before an attunement, even when they have never used Reiki before. I have even felt a good amount of Reiki coming out of people not interested in Reiki, including friends of mine who have nothing to do with my classes. Once you become able to perceive the Reiki energy you will find it commonly resides among ordinary people because the ability is not given from outside. In some cases, a good amount of Reiki starts to come out when one receives stimulus by watching something, going to a particular place or listening to something. These unintentionally improve one's Reiki flow in daily life. Another example of Reiki flow where no attunement is involved would be sitting in a Reiki circle for a while, a good amount of Reiki always comes out even after the circle is finished. These things happen because Reiki is an innate ability. The more I have taught, the more I have witnessed that Reiki is an ability commonly found in everyone. In this context, the idea of spiritual lineage is total nonsense, even harmful if you think of the negative ways people could use the idea.

Few people in Japan care about lineage, but all Western Reiki teachers abroad are concerned about their lineage and how close they are to Master Usui. A teacher is deemed to be bogus if he or she doesn't provide evidence of lineage.

The fact that everyone possesses the ability to do Reiki renders the idea of lineage meaningless. How and how much one practices is of far more importance. This is all Reiki practitioners should care about. If you think your ability was given to you by your teacher, you would of course become concerned about who gave them the ability, and so on. In the end, this concept of lineage can result in alarming discrimination! Though Western Reiki has many good features, the worst and most disturbing part is this idea of lineage.

I have often heard people talking of being superior or inferior depending on their lineage being closer or further away from Usui. I have also heard people talking of having an unclear lineage and how bad this is. If one thinks like this, it is more likely to degrade one's spirituality than assist it!

This idea of the inflated importance of lineage has come about because of the misconception that Reiki ability is given by others.

### The symbols

In Western Reiki a student can only use a particular symbol if he or she receives a certain attunement with that symbol. The symbols (I'm talking about the symbol and mantra when I say symbols here) are treated as sacred by many practitioners to the point that they feel powerless if they can't use them. Some teachers even believe the Reiki ability is activated by the symbols, making them play the most important, sacred role in Reiki. This is a delusion created once again by the simple but vital misunderstanding about where Reiki comes from. This delusion creates a morbid dependency on the symbols as in this mindset, without them one would become powerless.

In Japanese Reiki, symbols (to be precise they are known as shirushi and jumon) are mere tools used as supplements during treatments and the ability to use them is totally separate from the Reiju (done where Western Reiki has attunements). *I will say again, Reiki is an innate ability within everyone and this ability is not connected to the symbols.*

## The symbols - culture

In Japanese Reiki, it is easy to see that the shirushi and jumon have been created from the Japanese culture. They are not something mysterious, in fact they make sense and can be clearly understood in terms of Japan's cultural background.

In Western Reiki, people often find the symbols strange and difficult to understand. Without placing them in the context of cultural background, a teacher can easily make students believe in the symbols as mysterious and beyond their comprehension.

## The symbols - dependency leads to addiction

Once practitioners think Reiki ability comes from the symbols, they tend to depend heavily on them and start using them on virtually anything, often unable to do anything without them. In an effort to produce stronger and stronger effects, people come up with increasingly complex combinations of the symbols. I call this *symbol addiction*. It's a striking phenomenon observed in Western Reiki.

Some teachers even create entirely new symbols and use them to advertise their schools. In addition, many schools teach level 1 and level 2 over consecutive days, or even in a single day. The symbols are taught in level 2 so when students are taught so quickly they lack experience of using Reiki without the symbols and begin to think that it's not possible without them. Often, Reiki teachers, misunderstanding the use of symbols, think they are all they need to teach. This seriously degrades the quality of

Western Reiki schools and it all comes from that basic misunderstanding I've been talking about:

*Ignorance of one's natural ability* → *dependency on the symbols* → *degeneration of school quality*

This is one of the worst problems in the Western Reiki community.

In Japanese Reiki, the usage of shirushi and jumon are quite simple because the most important part of Reiki is achieved through one's own natural ability.

### Attunements Vs Reiju

Western Reiki teachers think the attunement in a given seminar level 'activates' a specific energy level of a student. For example, the attunement in level 1 activates the level-1 energy of a student and that in level 2 activates the level-2 energy of a student. So, the attunement differs in each seminar level. Western Reiki attunements are thought to 'upgrade' the student's energy level. This concept again comes from the misunderstanding of Reiki power as being given from outside.

In Japanese Reiki, there is only a single kind of Reiju. Given that Reiki is an innate ability, you may wonder why Reiju is needed at all. The amount of Reiki that naturally flows in each person depends on their physical, mental and emotional condition. The amount of Reiki initially flowing in a given person may not be enough to give an effective treatment. One can improve this Reiki flow by oneself through practicing Gokai or Hatsurei-ho without Reiju, but it needs effort and takes time. The Reiju improves the flow almost instantly without effort, just like cleaning a dirty or clogged pipe. Therefore, it is advantageous to use both of these. Reiju will clean your 'pipe' but it is your own self-cultivation - practicing Gokai in your daily life and Hatsurei-ho - that will make the pipe bigger.

Because the Reiju is simply 'cleaning a clogged pipe' it is always the same in Shoden, Okuden and even in Shinpiden. There is no such thing as level-1 or level-2 initiations. There is not even a Master initiation in Japanese Reiki.

According to the research by Robert Fueston described in his *The History and System of Usui Shiki Reiki Ryoho* (ISBN: 0997026804), Takata did not give the Master initiation to her early master students. He suspects Takata invented it for her later master students. This is probably true because there was and is no Master initiation in Japanese Reiki.

### *Controlling the flow Vs natural flow*

Many people misunderstand how Reiki comes out. In Western Reiki the misunderstanding about Reiki flowing naturally has caused people to think they have to make an effort to make Reiki flow in a certain way, using symbols or ceremonies. However, since Reiki is not something to be drawn out intentionally, it comes out of our hands (as well as certain other body parts) by itself when we are in a natural state. Some amount is even continuously coming out when we're relaxed. This is what I call, 'stationary

Reiki'. If we are tense, worried, angry or in a condition far from Gokai, the amount of Reiki flowing decreases.

When we apply our hands on someone, the amount of Reiki increases from the 'stationary level' according to the need in the receiver's body. If a hand is on a healthy part of the body, the amount of Reiki coming out will be more than when 'stationary', but not the most it can be. If the same hand is moved to an area that has a problem, the amount of Reiki flowing increases as shown in the illustration. We, as the practitioner, have absolutely no control over this flow. Reiki comes out at a greater rate

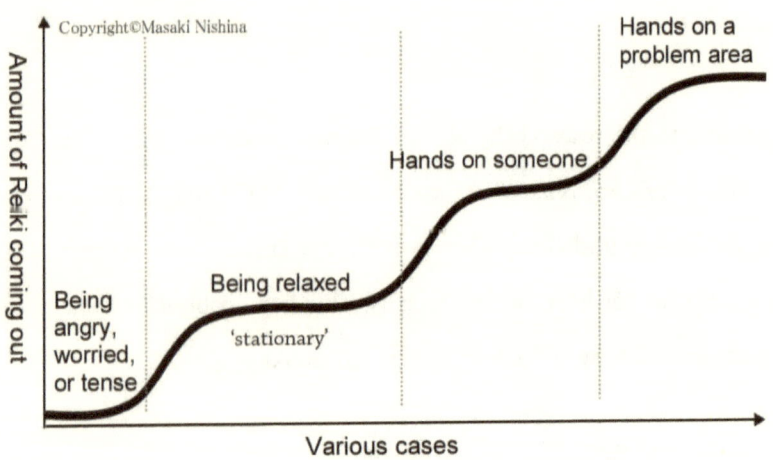

because it is being absorbed by cells and tissue that need to repair and revitalize - this area is depleted of energy and therefore automatically sucks Reiki from the hand. For this reason, the practitioner does not have to worry about drawing or pushing Reiki out, the only concern she or he has is WHERE to put the hand. This important knowledge was lost when the hand positions, in which practitioners spend only a short time in pre-determined positions (that may not even be problem areas) became so emphasized in Western Reiki.

The amount of Reiki coming out at any given time is also dependent on the size of the Reiki channel (or pipe) in your body. If you have a bigger or clearer pipe, the problem area in the receiver can absorb Reiki from it more easily. A Reiki beginner may not have a clear or big pipe compared to an experienced practitioner, but this does not mean it won't work as well for the beginner, it simply means they must put their hands on the area for a longer time. The total amount is more important than the speed at which it goes in. This is the reason even a total beginner can use Reiki effectively.

You may remember in Chapter 2 I talked about Usui treating a woman with a lower back problem who had not been able to stand up for a year. He treated her for 20-30 minutes and she was able to stand up and start to walk. His Reiki was not special or different from others, it's just that his 'pipe' was bigger and clearer and she was able to receive a great deal of Reiki in a short period of time. Other practitioners could help her to do the same, it would simply take longer.

As you can see, when practitioners are giving Reiki there is little they can do, other than relax and let go, to change the flow of the energy - it's a natural process. However, they can improve their capacity to flow the energy over time. In the Western idea of Reiki, this is thought to be done instantaneously by adding things on from the outside in the form of symbols etc., but in Japanese Reiki it is known that the most powerful way to increase one's capacity to flow Reiki energy is through self-cultivation

(Gokai, looking within rather than outside, Hatsurei-ho, living in harmony with nature etc.). You may recall from an earlier chapter that the importance of self-cultivation through Gokai is written on Usui's memorial stone.

## Ceremonial techniques

Thinking Reiki ability is given from outside us leads to a belief that there is something we have to do to start or activate it, which makes sense if we are not normally connected to Reiki. Some Reiki schools teach that students cannot use Reiki without first performing ceremonies such as Reiki shower or Reiki prayer. In reality of course, these are not necessary to start a Reiki treatment. We can use Reiki anytime, anywhere without having to push a 'start' button!

In Japanese Reiki ceremonies are not mandatory. However, our consciousness is not perfect and so ceremonies can help with clearing the mind and reducing anxiety. If one can't believe in oneself, ceremonies can help - this is a good part of Western Reiki. If you like to use them, use them. Be warned though, that once they become mandatory, they create unnecessary anxiety and harm one's own ability as a result. I teach Western Reiki students that Reiki is an innate ability and so for them the ceremonial techniques are totally unnecessary because they know Reiki is always with them.

## Degrees of freedom

You may assume that Western Reiki offers more freedom than Japanese

Reiki. It is probably true to some extent, but not so much as you may think. Many Western Reiki schools teach various rules and contraindications that bind the hands and feet of the practitioners who are warned either that terrible things will happen if they *do* a certain thing, or that terrible things will happen if they *don't do* a certain thing. I can list a dozen of them which would make Japanese Reiki practitioners laugh. It is very interesting, even ironic that Western Reiki, developed in democratic countries has fewer degrees of freedom than Japanese Reiki, birthed in pre-war Japan.

In Japanese Reiki, one's intuition plays an important role. For example, a practitioner perceives Byosen to find problematic parts when treating a client. Reiji-ho (mentioned in Chapter 9) is a further intuitive method to find problematic areas (this is not taught in Jikiden Reiki). The treatments in Japanese Reiki are not bound by formats or rules.

*Standardized framework*

When I looked into Western Reiki I started to realize American people generally tend to prefer something given to them in a format, something standardized. The strategy of chain stores like McDonald's is a good example of this. They have the same standard merchandise and service in every store, all controlled by a single 'how-to' manual.

In the US, each person has a significantly different level of education, amount of knowledge and ability to learn. People come from a wide variety of economic, racial and cultural backgrounds each with their own perceptions on life. In such an environment, making things standardized does ensure the quality of products and service. This may well be the background for the standard hand positions that became so popular in Western Reiki.

Conversely, Japanese people prefer service to be adaptable and thoughtful. In Japan this is known as *O-motenashi*. The person serving observes each customer carefully and thoughtfully, then adjusts his or her service to the customer - the very opposite of McDonald's. Japanese people are often misunderstood as being entirely uniform, probably because they tend to want to have a shared experience with others. They feel safe having things in common and insecure in being different. Shinto emphasizes harmony among people as well. However, all this does not mean Japanese people prefer things uniform and standardized. In fact, they place a high value on things intuitive and adaptable.

Since the occupation, sadly many Japanese are so Americanized that it is possible to see the same phenomenon of standardization in Japan as in America. There are about 3,000 McDonald's shops in Japan now! And there are now many Western Reiki schools that teach McDonald-ized Reiki.

### Reiki teachers

The system to create teachers in Western Reiki is very different from that in Japanese Reiki. In Western Reiki one can become a Reiki 'teacher' even if one is very inexperienced. Many schools issue teacher certificates to people who simply sit in a seminar room for a day, with no continuous training or examination. The certificate is basically given as an exchange for an expensive seminar fee. These 'teachers' are often called 'masters' which is nonsensical and shameful for the Reiki community. They are using the word 'master' erroneously. A teacher does not make someone else a master. A 'master initiation' does not make someone a master. A piece of paper that states someone is a master does not make it so. The state of being master can be only reached by achievement with one's daily efforts, self-cultivation and with considerable respect from others.

There are quite a number of Reiki schools run by 'masters' who have no ability to teach. Furthermore, some schools teach levels 1, 2, 3 and the teacher level in a very short period of time. In the worst case, a single day! There is even a business run on the internet that issues a 'teacher' certificate if one sends an application with money - it's unbelievable.

Western Reiki has evolved into such an unsound system that it creates many irresponsible teachers. Such teachers go on to create the next generation of irresponsible teachers and so the quality diminishes further over time. It is in quite a state and I think should be seen unfavorably by the general public as well as those within it. There are no excuses for this kind of unprincipled, immoral system of producing Reiki teachers. This is another of the worst problems facing the Western Reiki community today.

The Japanese system of creating teachers is based on that of traditional martial arts and *Do*, such as Judo, Kendo or Sado. One can become shihan-kaku (assistant teacher) if, and only if, one accumulates enough experience in treating many clients. A candidate typically spends more than a year to become shihan-kaku. He or she can become shihan (teacher) only when enough experience teaching as shihan-kaku has been gained. When learning anything in Japan, everyone naturally follows such a system as an unwritten rule. It's part of Japanese culture. Jikiden Reiki follows this and allows only dai-shihan (senior teachers) to create shihan-kaku. Only two people, the representative and vice-representative are able to create shihans. In this way, the desired quality of teachers is maintained.

### Is Japanese Reiki more powerful?

Some Jikiden Reiki practitioners advertise their Reiki as being more powerful than Western Reiki. I believe that using such an expression is foolish. However, I can imagine the reasons behind their claims.

If one's mind is more calm and peaceful, more Reiki will flow. The flow can be blocked or reduced if one has a lot of anxiety or anger. The more you practice Gokai (The five principles) the more Reiki will flow. As I mentioned before, in typical Western Reiki systems, the excess use of ceremonial techniques and the contraindications can cause anxiety if, for example, people wonder if they are really connected to Reiki or whether they have done the procedures adequately. They may be worrying, "Did I forget something?", or, "Am I doing anything wrong?" during a treatment. All these result in the reduction of Reiki flow.

A second reason is that there are quite a number of Western Reiki teachers who are incapable of teaching and performing an attunement properly because they have not been taught well themselves. Their attunements and classes may not be good enough to adequately improve Reiki flow in students. I have met many such students who first learned Western Reiki in other schools and then came to mine because they could not understand or use Reiki.

For these reasons people sometimes mistakenly think that Western Reiki isn't as good. On the contrary, Western Reiki is very effective if one learns it correctly.

## Now/today Vs past/future

Japanese Reiki deals only with *now and today* as suggested in the Gokai. To worry about what has already happened is pointless because the past cannot be changed. To overcome something from the past, we need only deal with what is present now and today. In doing this, we change the future because the future is created by what we are doing and being now and today. That is Japanese Reiki.

In Western Reiki however, people try to heal the past and send Reiki energy into the future. When we are trapped in the past, we attribute our problem to karma, trauma, environment, or sometimes the actions of parents or others. This may help us to feel psychologically relieved but will not solve our problems. In the West people believe causality is very important in solving problems. While that is an effective approach in scientific research, it is not necessarily so in solving personal problems because we are simply attributing the problem to something out of our control. To think, "I'm not the one causing my problems," is to postpone solving the problems by placing responsibility on something uncontrollable.

In Japanese Reiki, every human possesses the wonderful ability to solve his or her own problems his or herself without handing over the responsibility to others or the past.

Some Western Reiki schools make claims in their advertisements such as, "Our Reiki seminar will change your life to a happy one." Surprisingly, a number of people are attracted by this kind of advertisement. However, if one is in a vulnerable mental state and is unable to solve personal problems then Western Reiki offers helpful and heart-warming techniques such as healing the past, sending Reiki to the future and wish fulfillment.

### DKM - The Western Reiki symbol

It may come as a surprise to you but the fourth symbol (DKM), which is taught as a 'master symbol' in the third level of Western Reiki, does not and has never existed in Japanese Reiki. Many schools teach DKM as the most important symbol and treat it as something sacred and absolute. This symbol - or the lack of it - is the fundamental difference between Japanese and Western Reiki. In this section I'm going to look at what DKM really is, provide reasons and evidence to show that it has never existed in Japanese Reiki and suggest where it may have come from.

*DKM - What is it?*

Firstly, let's take a clear look at how DKM is taught in typical Western Reiki schools.

- DKM is called the master symbol.
- DKM often supersedes other symbols.
- DKM is omnipotent and an all-purpose enhancement.
- DKM promotes harmony and the evolution of the universe.
- DKM symbolizes the entire universe and enlightenment.
- DKM improves one's spirituality.
- DKM guides one to enlightenment.

That is to say, DKM is an absolute super symbol. When I first learned the third level of Western Reiki, DKM made me feel very uncomfortable because it seemed religious.

If I tell Western Reiki practitioners that DKM did not originally exist in Reiki they are often so shocked it seems as though their world has been turned upside down. This illustrates the sacredness, even absoluteness it is given in the West. When Frank Arjava Petter tried to publish his book, *This is Reiki* in which he provides evidence that DKM didn't exist in original Japanese Reiki, his publisher delayed publication for two years because it was thought the information would have such adverse effects on the Western Reiki community!

Secondly, let's look at what DKM is to Japanese.

- DKM is nothing special to an educated Japanese person.

- DKM consists of three plain kanji characters written in a column.

- DKM 's KM is an ordinary word meaning *enlightenment.*

- DKM 's combination of kanji is not something you need to learn in an expensive seminar.

- DKM is used in the names of some Buddhist sects.

- DKM is not a technique and can only be seen as such by non-Japanese who do not know kanji.

As a geometric figure DKM is not special, only three ordinary kanji characters, D, K, and M. The first, D, means *great* or *big.* The second 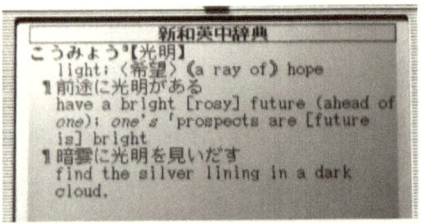 and third, KM, together mean *enlightenment.* KM is a word often used in Buddhism, it's in the name of some Buddhist sects and is also an ordinary word known to educated Japanese people. It is in any ordinary dictionary as shown in the picture. Hence, it is not a special technique and not something a person needs to pay to learn!

Teaching DKM to non-Japanese people is the equivalent of teaching the phrase, 'Great Enlightenment' to non-English speaking people as a technique to lead them to enlightenment. Imagine telling someone, "Writing and chanting the words, 'Great Enlightenment' will definitely bring you enlightenment!"

The three kanji characters used in DKM are simply arranged in a column, not fused together like the kanji in the third symbol HSZSN. For non-Japanese people it is difficult to distinguish a graphical symbol from a word made from kanji but DKM is definitely not a graphical symbol. It would be very strange if after making the other three symbols original graphic creations, Usui suddenly made the most important 'master' symbol nothing but an ordinary kanji word. If you were Japanese, you would feel something was amiss.

Interestingly however, when young Japanese people learn DKM, some receive it as something extraordinary, like Western people do. They lack traditional Japanese knowledge. The effect of Westernization is so large.

*DKM - evidence it never existed in Japanese Reiki*

In Japanese Reiki, it is important to cultivate one's mind and improve one's spirituality through the practice of Gokai. Everyone has wonderful potential and abilities so persistent effort leads to wonderful things. Self-reliance, in which we are the source of our own salvation, is the important idea Japanese Reiki teaches us. The idea of using DKM is part of the Western mindset of dependency on others. It is the exact opposite of what Japanese Reiki is teaching.

Having learned the first level, students have precious experiences and begin to improve their spirituality through practice of the Gokai. They will realize the wonderful ability they were born with and discover the shining possibility that they can improve themselves through their own efforts. To then introduce DKM which causes them to depend on something external would spoil all this at the last stage. It makes no sense unless one wants to make Reiki a religion. If Usui had taught DKM in prewar Japan, his students would have found it so absurd that he would have lost all the trust he had earned. At best, they may have thought he had created a new religion.

There are two pieces of clear evidence that DKM did not exist in Japanese Reiki.

(1) A student of Frank Arjava Petter had an interview with Fumio Ogawa, shihan (teacher) in Usui Reiki Ryoho Gakkai, in 1997. Once Ogawa had confirmed that three symbols (one is a jumon but I have used the word symbol for ease of reference here) are used in Japanese Reiki, she asked Ogawa about DKM. The following is an excerpt from the description on page 262-263 of Petter's *This is Reiki*.

*Question*: How many symbols do you use? What do they look like and where do they originate?

*Answer*: The first symbol comes from Shintoism, and the second is a bonji (Sanskrit seed syllable). The third is a shortened conglomeration of five Kanji, a Jumon (magical formula) (author/interviewer's note: I had asked Shizuko to show him the symbols that are commonly used abroad, and he agreed with them, more or less.)

*Question*: What about the Master Symbol? (Shizuko writes it and show it to him.)

*Answer.* I have never seen that before.

(2) *Mamoru Doi*, a member of Usui Reiki Ryoho Gakkai, writes on page 129 of his book "*Reiki: Energy filling the universe*" (published only in Japanese) :

If we compare the symbols in Western Reiki and traditional Japanese Reiki, they are not perfectly identical but very much alike. ........ I do not mention anything about the fourth symbol to avoid confusion.

He clearly means there is something odd about the fourth symbol, DKM. In addition on page 162 to 163, he writes:

In Western Reiki, people have the tenacious thought, 'To live one's life positively, Reiki should be used for self-improvement and wish fulfillment.' ......Other than the Gokai, the Reiki treatment they learned lacks concrete know-how that brings peace of mind. To reach their goals, they developed the meditation and methods of wish-fulfillment, and further introduced the fourth symbol that would connect them to something holy.

Therefore, Doi implicitly admits the fourth symbol, DKM, was newly introduced when Western Reiki was developed.

In summary, there is no evidence that DKM was used in Japanese Reiki and all the information we have indicates that it was not. It sends students in the opposite direction than the self-cultivation of Japanese Reiki and it is not taught in Japanese Reiki seminars.

*DKM - Where did it come from?*

DKM is a Western technique developed in the Western community by somebody who knew a little about the Japanese language. It may well be Takata who introduced DKM when she invented a 'master initiation' for a later group of her master students though it could have happened somewhere else along the line of her students. For them, DKM is very much like an idol to worship. It symbolizes Western Reiki and is the key that differentiates Western and Japanese Reiki. In short, *if one teaches DKM, it is Western Reiki.*

Whoever introduced this symbol understood the characteristics of Western people well and had great foresight. It plays an important role in Western Reiki. It even works fairly effectively in Westernized Japan at present too. DKM helps people who don't have confidence in themselves, dislike longterm persistent effort and have dependency on others. Whoever writes and chants it may become happier, more or less, and it is ok to use if it is effective for you.

There are two possible religious groups in Japan that someone may have taken the idea of DKM from. Both groups use the three letters DKM for the God they worship. The first is *Sekai Kyusei Kyo* (世界救世教). They are famous for their hands-on healing. They worship 'DKM真神', where 真 means true and 神 means God. The second is *Kurama Ko Kyo* (鞍馬弘教), the group I mentioned in Chapter 3 when talking about Mt Kurama. They worship Sonten (尊天) which represents the great spirit, great enlightenment (DKM), and great active body of the universe.

These may not be connected but there is the possibility that a Western person familiar enough with Japanese culture to know the hands-on healing group or Kurama Ko Kyo, introduced DKM into Western Reiki. Wherever it came from, it is important to know that DKM has nothing to with Japanese Reiki.

## *Evolving spiritually Vs evolving tools*

The question of whether spiritual or technical evolution is more important illustrates another difference between Japanese and Western Reiki.

Shinto is hugely influential in Japanese life. I started to learn Shinto when I was studying the cultural background of Japanese Reiki. I was surprised to find that Shinto deeply affects our everyday lives and values in Japan, far more than I had thought. Many Japanese would not be able to explain what Shinto is well, yet their lives are affected by it in some way every day. Shinto may be the embodiment of Japanese culture - or Japanese culture may embody Shinto, or perhaps it is both.

One such influence Shinto has endowed on Japanese culture is the tendency to try to evolve oneself rather than to use technology to evolve tools. According to Shinto philosophy, the purpose of one's life is to raise oneself (in the sense of bringing up a child) and improve one's spirituality, which places a higher value on self-improvement than improving techniques. In Western Reiki, techniques seem to be the leading characteristics because power is thought to reside outside, while in Japanese Reiki, techniques are supplemental and humans are the leading characters because the real power resides within.

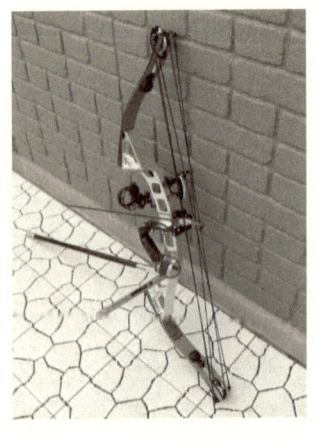

*Kyudo Vs archery*

The comparison of Kyudo and archery is a good example of this contrast. As you can see in the picture, an archery bow is an accumulation of various technologies. It is made of hi-tech carbon fiberglass and is armed with many mechanical adjustments for balancing and targeting. The bow has been improved in such a way as to obtain a better hitting rate. One's personal skill is important of course, but the tool plays an essential part in the process. This archery bow reminds me of how symbols/mantras are used in Western Reiki. The purpose of archery is to hit a target as a sport, in competition or as a hobby.

On the other hand, the purpose of Kyudo (弓道, the way of the bow) is connected to Shinto. A Kyudo practitioner may want to hit the target, but that is not his or her underlying purpose. This bow is made of bamboo and

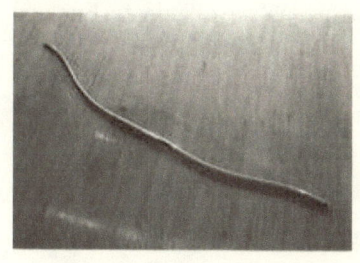 uses hemp strings and rattan. The design has essentially remained unchanged for 400 years. Traditional Japanese tools are generally simple, often made of wood, paper, bamboo, hemp and soil (ceramic). This doesn't mean Japanese people are undeveloped, primitive or behind in some way. On the contrary, in the world of *do* such as Kyudo, Kendo (剣道, the way of the sword), Shodo (書道, the way of writing), Judo (柔道, the way of flexibility) and Sado (茶道, the way of tea), the purpose is to improve personal skill and spirituality. It is not to improve tools.

As I have said, Shinto (神道, the way of god) teaches that the purpose of life is to improve one's spirituality, therefore, in Kyudo it would be meaningless to get a better hitting rate just by improving tools because it 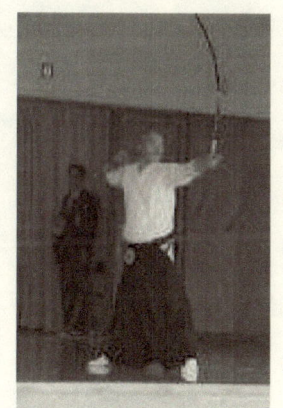 has nothing to do with one's spirituality. Of course the desire is to improve one's hitting rate, but it should be achieved through one's own skill and level of spirituality rather than by employing technology. This is what *do* (道, the way) is. If a Kyudo practitioner and an archery practitioner have the same level of skill, the archery practitioner would probably yield a better hitting rate. In Western thinking the Kyudo practitioner would be judged as inferior but in Japanese thinking, though they are the same in terms of skill, the Kyudo practitioner may well have more spiritual alignment.

For those interested in Shinto, I recommend a book available in English, *The Essence of Shinto: Japan's Spiritual Heart* written by Motohisa Yamakage (ISBN: 1568364377)

If you apply what I have explained here to Japanese and Western Reiki, you can see how one is linked to spiritual evolution, and the other is clearly focussed on tools and technical evolution.

### The value of Western Reiki and Japanese Reiki

Western Reiki kindly helps people who are mentally weakened or have lost confidence while Japanese Reiki encourages people to be strong and self-reliant.

If one is brought up being told they are powerless and come from original sin, needing to be saved by God, one would most likely feel weakened and lose confidence in themselves. Conversely, if one is brought up being told that they are branched off from the great existence and have the potential for wonderful power, one would most likely feel strong and self-reliant.

As I mention in the early parts of this book, after the defeat of the war and the occupation, Japanese people have come to grow up in an atmosphere of self-denial where they are treated more as weak, low class, inferior and behind. I have observed how many people have lost their bearings, obsessed with their karma and trauma. They are trapped in their past and worry about their future. In this context, it would be obvious that Japanese would be attracted by Western Reiki, offering something good from outside. Nowadays a great many people both in Japan and the West crave healing and salvation. They may feel they cannot be as strong as Japanese Reiki teaches. In situations such as this, Western Reiki is probably what people need.

Western Reiki can be widely applied to many aspects of daily life using a variety of techniques with a flexible curriculum. However, the contents of Japanese Reiki should be maintained and succeeded to future generations as a precious inheritance. We need a separate framework in order to develop new applications that accommodate the new age. While I continue to teach Jikiden Reiki with a solid fixed curriculum, I make full use of Western Reiki because I can adjust and optimize the seminar contents for each student's need. We need both.

In my Western Reiki class, I teach people about Reiki not being given from outside, I teach them how Reiki is an ability that everyone possesses when they are born. Once people fully understand this correction, the parts of Western Reiki adversely affected by Western culture automatically diminish and Western Reiki is free to provide advantages that Japanese Reiki doesn't. I am able to do this because I have learned Jikiden Reiki and observed the differences.

## Summary

Below is a summary of all the Japanese techniques I have mentioned in this book that have been removed during the evolution of Western Reiki and the additions made as Western Reiki became what it is today. I'm referring here to the modern Western Reiki rather than Takata's teachings I described in Chapter 9. You will see that there are some good additions in Western Reiki, but equally some important things have been lost.

## *Summary of techniques removed*

### *Clinical techniques*

- Perceiving Byosen
- Shirushi on Byosen
- Blood circulation method
- Tanden detoxification

It is ironic that these techniques are listed as the most important techniques in a brochure published by Usui Reiki Ryoho Gakkai.

### *Intuitive techniques*

- Perceiving Byosen
- Reiji method

Western people seem to prefer non-intuitive standardized techniques. They seem to dislike learning such intuitive techniques.

### *Self-improvement techniques*

- Hatsu-rei ho
- Stress on self-cultivation
- Importance of Gokai

Hatsu-rei ho is a meditation-like method that improves one's Reiki flow. Western people seem to prefer instant results without long-term self training.

## Kotodama

Kotodama means the spirit of language or the miraculous power of language. It is different from mantra. The power of kotodama has been utilized since ancient times in Japan, of course not only in Reiki but in a wide variety of fields. Japanese Reiki uses several kotodama, all of which have been lost in Western Reiki, including Gokai. Although Gokai has been translated into English for Western Reiki the power of the original sound was lost. It is probably inevitable that kotodama would be lost when teaching in a different language. Takata probably did not understand how kotodama works.

## Summary of techniques _added_

### Aura and chakras

The clinical techniques have been substituted by healing methods such as treating the aura and chakras. This results in a more pleasant and soothing treatment than Japanese Reiki.

### Soothing attunements

Reiju became _attunement_ in Western Reiki. As a technique, they are similar but they have some differences. While Reiju gives a powerful impression, a good attunement provides a very pleasant, soothing, comfortable and peaceful feeling. The attunement employs various techniques that create such feelings. I think it is unfortunate if you have only experienced Reiju because a good attunement feels so good!

*Standardized techniques*

- Standard hand positions (12 hand positions)
- Mandatory use of ceremonial methods
- Mandatory use of aura purification
- Mandatory 21-day self-healing
- Various contraindications

Western people seem to like shoulds and shouldn'ts. They seem to care quite considerably about getting things right and not being wrong. Many Western Reiki teachers like to teach various contraindications and rules which are actually totally unnecessary.

*External dependence*

- Sanctification of symbols and mantras
- The fourth symbol, the Master symbol (DKM)
- Complex use of symbols and mantras
- Ceremonial methods to 'start' Reiki

These are the very characteristics of Western Reiki. They tend to borrow external powers without making use of one's own power through practice, training and experience.

*Techniques for peace of mind*

- Extended use of the second symbol (SHK)
- The fourth symbol, the Master symbol (DKM)
- Techniques for wish fulfillment

In the developed countries where Western Reiki became popular, many people are under considerable mental stress and suffer from psychological problems. For those people, these techniques are very helpful, especially the extended use of the second symbol SHK, which allows a healer to use the energy of affection and mercy during a healing session. The second symbol is effective in mental healing, giving the receiver a sense of deep relaxation and peace of mind.

*Spiritual teachings*

- The third level seminar
- The fourth symbol, the Master symbol (DKM)

The third level Western Reiki seminar teaches spiritual techniques said to help gain enlightenment, to communicate with a higher dimension, and to live one's life with confidence and peace of mind. Japanese Reiki, however, does not have a dedicated seminar that teaches concrete methods to improve one's spirituality other than practicing Gokai, where it is left to self-discipline and effort. Frankly speaking it is impossible to teach enlightenment in a seminar, but I think it is very good for a student to work on such subjects as part of a curriculum. This is a good part of Western Reiki.

*Departure from now and today*

- Healing the past
- Sending Reiki to the future
- Wish fulfillment

Western people like to search out the cause of something and clarify the relationship between cause and result. Such a tendency sometimes leads to excessive worry about the past and future. It may be human nature to be trapped in the past or become anxious about the future. Western Reiki offers techniques to ease worry and fulfill wishes.

## Widened application

- Reiki for pets
- Reiki for human relationships
- Reiki for situations

All these techniques have been created to accommodate the wishes of modern people. Before the war, especially in Japan, there was no concept of 'pets', they were just domestic animals. After the war, animals became more like family members. It is also natural to apply Reiki for human relationships or difficult situations because people often worry about them.

## Disordered and irresponsible teaching system

There are many Western Reiki schools that:

- teach each level in very short time (e.g. a few hours)
- teach three levels in a short period (e.g. a month)
- teach the first and second level in a day
- teach all three levels in a day
- give a teacher-level seminar to an inexperienced student
- teach all three levels and the teacher level in a day
- give little hands-on practice during a seminar
- give a teacher certificate to an inexperienced student

Some Western Reiki teachers and practitioners appear to have lost their common sense. The general public have generally not, and so when they see these things happening they naturally assume Western Reiki to be irresponsible and immoral. Unfortunately, there is no easy way to regulate the behaviour of these schools and teachers.

The tendency to teach advanced classes a very short period of time after the first level has even extended to Jikiden Reiki. In Tokyo and Osaka, Hayashi taught an Okuden (advanced) class separately from Shoden (first) class, typically a few months apart. He only taught them consecutively when teaching in remote areas, when he spent about five days in total on them. In the present Jikiden Reiki system, Shoden and Okuden are typically taught consecutively over only about two and a half days. I think this is unfortunate.

Such teaching schedules have been chosen for students' convenience and teachers' profit but it doesn't benefit a student's learning because Reiki is not knowledge. It is experience and practice. It is absolutely necessary for a student to practice Reiki sufficiently by him or herself after the first class, before taking the next level. I would have thought this to be common sense, however, it doesn't seem to be so in the Reiki community today. It is relevant to share one of the Meiji Emperor's poems here, posted at Meiji shrine. It says, "Everything has its best timing. Even knowing that, people unfortunately tend to walk too fast."

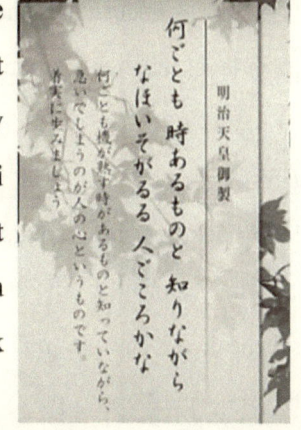

## How I teach my Western Reiki classes

Given that I have been critical of Western Reiki, you may wonder how I teach my Western Reiki classes. I'll share a little with you here.

Before teaching anything technical, I find it is very important to teach the following:

1. Reiki is an innate ability that everyone possesses from birth. It is not something given from outside.
2. We are connected to Reiki all the time and everywhere.
3. Reiki energy has no particular intentions. A recipient's body uses the energy for it's own purpose.
4. Reiki is the natural energy that flows out spontaneously when one is relaxed without intentions.
5. An affected area of the body absorbs a large amount of Reiki by itself. Don't try to send Reiki intentionally.

If a student understands these principles, the class goes nice and smoothly. Each level requires six hours and three attunements.

*Level 1*

I do not teach any ceremonial techniques or ways to 'start' Reiki because we are connected all the time. I teach the standard hand positions, self-healing, Hatsurei-ho, techniques to perceive Hibiki (equivalent to Byosen) and how to purify things and places. A student spends about half of the seminar time practicing hands-on.

*Level 2*

The symbols and mantras are introduced to enhance the effects and help healings. Again, a student spends about half of the seminar time on practicing the symbols/mantras.

I *never* teach two levels consecutively, even in Jikiden Reiki. A student spends more than two months after level 1 or Shoden before the next step. The minimum six-month practice is required after level 2 and prior to level 3.

*Level 3*

The fourth symbol, DKM, is introduced as a symbol that enhances one's receptivity so that one can use one's intuition more easily and connect to higher dimensions more smoothly. I do not place DKM above the other symbols. A student receives various trainings to enhance his or her five senses, and the sixth sense. I also teach Reiji-ho, methods to sense aura and chakras and techniques to read others intuitively.

Some Jikiden Reiki shihan-kaku and shihan are Western Reiki teachers at the same time. They often start having troubles in teaching Western Reiki after becoming shihan-kaku or shihan because the common Western Reiki contradicts Japanese Reiki, especially at level 3.

Change your teaching as shown above!

Western Reiki is very flexible after all, isn't it!

# Chapter 12  Other Surviving Alternative Therapies

Other therapies born before and during the war have survived and continue to be used today. Some have continued to advance. It's important to recognize and promote them as part of the wider healing Japan needs to go through since the cultural self-denial that happened after the war. I'll briefly introduce a few in this chapter.

## Nishi-shiki Health Management (西式健康法)

Katsuzo Nishi (西勝造) developed his health management system in 1927. Nishi-shiki methods to promote health and healing include:

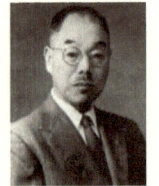

- a diet of fresh vegetables and brown rice
- alternate hot/cold bathing
- fasting
- physical exercise

As I described in Chapter 8, some people used this method along with Reiki. My father practiced Nishi-shiki methods when he was young and in 2011 I spent nine days at a Nishi-shiki school practicing fasting and the above methods. I believe this has vastly improved my digestive system. Recently, some medical doctors make use of Nishi-shiki methods to treat cancer patients quite effectively alongside radiation and chemotherapy.

## Macrobiotics

Macrobiotics has become fairly well-known across the world. Originally this dietary method was developed by Yukikazu Sakurazawa (桜沢如一 1893 - 1966, later known as *George Ohsawa* in the US) in pre-war Japan. He first learned about 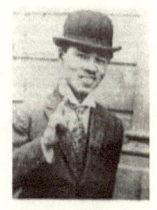 the importance of balanced diet from Sagen Ishizuka (石塚左玄 1851 - 1909) a doctor and a pharmacist during the Meiji era.

Sakurazawa's macrobiotic diet is based on brown rice as a staple food, with vegetables, pickles and dry foods included, similar to a traditional Japanese diet. In order to maintain nutritional balance, he introduced a yin yang theory into his system as well. Sakurazawa visited France in 1929 to promote macrobiotics abroad and in 1960, he moved to the US with his pupil, Michi Kushi (久司道夫 1926 - 2014). Together they presented macrobiotics as *Zen Macrobiotics*, using the philosophy and eating practices of Zen Buddhism, and it became very popular among the new age community. These days there are groups all over the world that have evolved from Sakurazawa's original system and quite a few macrobiotic restaurants as well as supermarkets or stores where one can buy prepared macrobiotic food.

## Oketani System of Breast-feeding (桶谷式母乳管理法)

http://www.oketani-kensankai.jp/html/eng.html

http://www.oketani-rso.com/

Sotomi Oketani (桶谷そとみ 1913 - 2004) created a unique breast-feeding system. Having worked as a nurse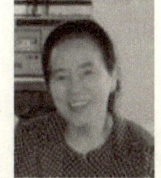

and midwife in Shinkyo (新京) the capital of Manchuria, during the war, she witnessed many babies dying due to the lack of their mother's milk. This led her to study how to enhance the mother's production of milk and she established her own system of breast-feeding based on her experience.

After being evacuated to Takaoka city in Japan, she opened a clinic and continued to refine her system based on the clinical experience she gained there. In 1974, she announced her system complete and introduced it publicly as the *Oketani system of breast-feeding*. Her method has gradually gained popularity among nurses and midwives.

Oketani's system is a total care system consisting of breast massage, diet recommendations and breast-feeding techniques. As part of her theory, she advocated that breastfeeding enhances the physical and mental condition of both mother and child.

This system is very helpful as many mothers have difficulty with breast-feeding. In fact, prior to my learning Reiki, both my ex-wife and my current wife followed Oketani's methods and found them invaluable. Because of this, I knew of the system, but only researched its history when I was studying the history of Japanese Reiki. I felt emotional when I realized that something originating in war-time Japan had helped my family so much.

To date, about a dozen Oketani practitioners have come to learn Reiki at my school and are now using Reiki to enhance their breast massage.

## Noguchi Seitai

Much of the *Seitai* (整体 regulating body) bodywork practiced these days originated from Noguchi Seitai. Haruchika Noguchi (野口晴哉 1911 - 1976) learned from a Reijutsu-ka, Doubetsu Matsumoto, and in 1926, at the tender 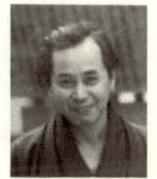 age of 15, he founded the *Institute for Natural Health Maintenance* in Iriya, Tokyo.

Noguchi established his Seitai method both by studying various therapies around the world and through his own research. The word *Seitai* is his creation. He believed illness and disease come from *Tai heki* (体癖 body habits) which are acquired in one's daily life. His methods include self-regulating practice to break the body habits, regulation of the spinal column and the hands-on therapy called *Yuki* described in Chapter 3.

## Shiatsu (指圧 finger pressure)

The *Shiatsu* therapy practiced nowadays is thought to have been established by Tokujiro Namikoshi (浪越徳治郎, 1905 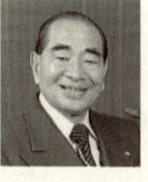 - 2000) around 1920. Shiatsu promotes the client's self-healing process by pushing vital points on the body. Namikoshi, and the word Shiatsu, became very famous after he treated Marilyn Monroe several times during her visit to Japan in 1954.

Please feel free to research these therapies more, or to try them for yourself!

# Chapter 13    Why Reiki Originated in Japan

If Reiki is a natural ability and simple enough that anyone can use it, why didn't something similar emerge from other countries?

There is a distinct inevitability to Reiki being birthed in Japan. In fact, it could *only* have been discovered in Japan. The reason is closely associated with the unique characteristics of traditional Japanese culture. In previous chapters I have defined many of the differences between the original Japanese Reiki and the Reiki we see today in the West. In this chapter, I'd like to look more closely at aspects of the two cultures to understand why it had to be Japan that gave birth to this miraculous healing energy therapy.

## Nature

The original Japanese culture was primarily characterized by the awareness of our co-existence and co-habitation with nature. Rather than taking advantage of nature purely as a physical 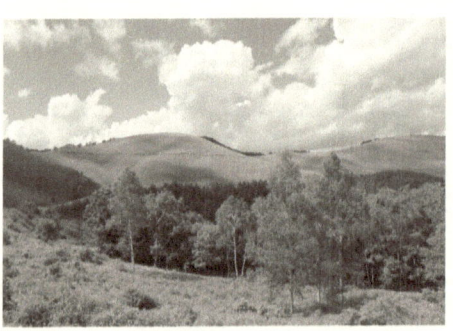 resource, people saw its infinite power and worked to co-exist with gratitude.

One of the most fundamental differences therefore between Japanese and Western culture is the presence or absence of *awe before nature*. The sense for Japanese is that there is an inestimable special power in nature, beyond human comprehension and that we must happily co-exist with this to live our lives. Until Western culture entered Japan, the Japanese people existed by virtue of nature, therefore they placed nature before

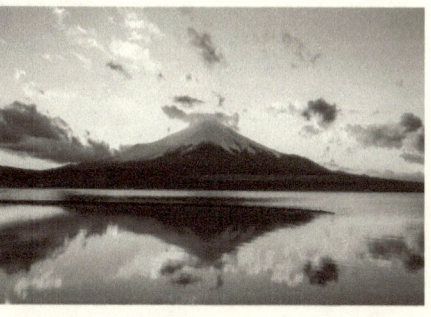

themselves. Gifts were harnessed from nature, but in a way that allowed for co-habitation. The Japanese lived entirely in this way, with a perfect ecosystem, until the beginning of Westernization in the Meiji era.

In the West, humans are placed at the center of the world, they tend to distinguish themselves from nature, unfamiliar with the level of awe the original Japanese culture holds. Because of this mindset, nature and the surrounding environment is simply something to benefit them. It's a physical resource to be controlled, utilized and taken advantage of. If it doesn't serve their purpose as it is, it is forcibly changed.

This contrast gives rise to diametrically opposed value systems in which one is integrating with nature by '*letting things be*' while the other is purposefully struggling to, '***bring things into being***' no matter the cost.

*Gardens*

In the West, generally, gardens are based on a shape and geometry not found in nature, while in Japan, even the artificial embodies a sense of awe before nature. A Japanese garden for example, is an artificial creation of

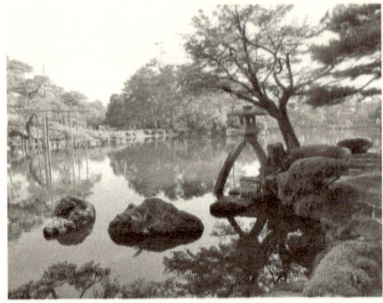 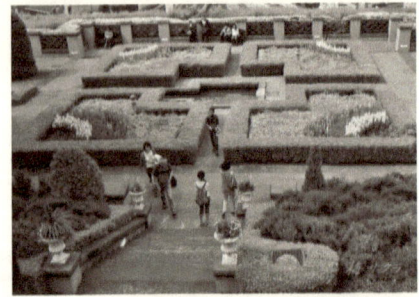

beauty in nature. Bonsai is a similar creation, in which the beauty and intricacy of trees are artificially replicated on a desktop. Any such artificial creation is infused with the Japanese profound reverence for nature.

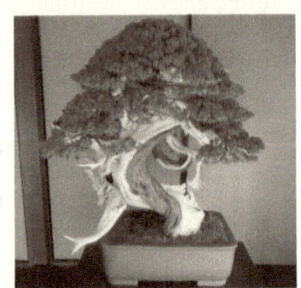

*Food*

Such awe is also found in Japanese food. Sushi for example, is seen as 'raw' in Western eyes, but to Japanese people, it is carefully, 'cooked'. The fish is not baked, boiled or fried but the

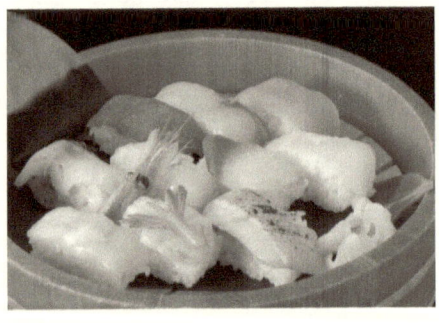

preparation, when done by a chef with the correct training, is both minimal and yet sophisticated. Because of this it is seen as 'cooked' in Japan. The materials used are simple, in as natural condition as possible and can seem primitive to those who don't understand. The intention, as with all Japanese food, is to unleash the exceptional in the taste of nature!

This concept is not generally seen in Western cooking.

## Housing

There was a time when Westerners would make fun of the Japanese, thinking them primitive and unsophisticated, comparing their small houses - made of wood, grass and paper - to rabbit hutches. If one looks more carefully though, it is possible to see just the opposite. House items in Japan are often examples of the very best craftsmanship. *Tatami* (Japanese flooring) is made of straw grass but it is a beautifully handcrafted object not seen elsewhere in the world. *Fusuma* and *shoji* (sliding doors) are also delicate pieces of artwork made from Japanese paper.

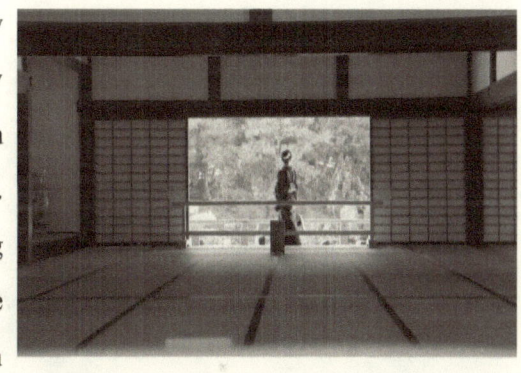

Though the size of houses usually matter greatly to Westerners, in Japan a 2m-by-2m space can represent an entire universe as seen in Sado (Tea Ceremony). This is another example of how Japanese live with nature. Rather than being primitive or uncultured, living in this way requires intelligence, patience, a sense of beauty and wisdom - all built on a 2,000 year old culture.

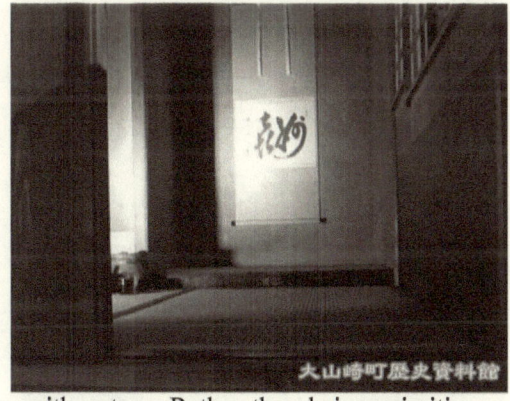

*Power*

For Japanese, the power contained in nature is essentially intrinsic in human as well. Living in harmony with nature allows us to exert a power equivalent to that of the nature of which we are in awe. Therefore, the more we are integrated with nature, the more we can use its wonderful power.

Western people tend to think humans remain powerless if they leave their lives to nature or 'let it be'. They often equate 'letting it be' with resignation. However, this ancient Japanese way of thinking is far from resignation, it's actually a way of tapping into the greatest source of power available. ***Reiki is an example of the power of 'letting it be'.***

**God and creation**

The Western idea of being so separate from nature is partly due to biblical concepts. The Bible teaches that the world was created by 'one God'. We must believe in that God, who created nature, rather than believe in the power of nature itself. Here, God exists above all and nature is a mere piece of God's work. The great event of creation in the Bible indicates there is a distinct cause of everything, therefore someone must have ***brought it into being.***

Japanese believe there are many Gods (kami), who created the Japanese Archipelago, but there is no concept of one God who created the world. To the Japanese mind, the world was not created, there was no cause or result, it naturally formed and it continues to exist in a flow of daily life. Therefore nature was not brought into being, it was there from the beginning. Nature is *being*.

*These concepts of 'brought into being' and 'being' have a great bearing on Reiki because **Reiki is not to be 'brought into being', instead Reiki is NATURALLY BEING.** Hence, everyone can do it.*

When humans are seen as separate from God, they are helpless, waiting to be salvaged from original sin. In such a culture one would hardly believe that every person is endowed with the advanced ability to heal people. This is why practitioners of Western Reiki often think that we are incapable of performing Reiki until we are granted some special ability from outside. It is also understandable that they would think we need to activate Reiki every time we use it through some special procedure - since we are not normally connected. Such thinking then undeniably originates from biblical cultures where people are taught to believe in God but not themselves.

You are most likely familiar with Star Wars, the US science fiction movie in which the characters hold special powers. They are often heard to say, "*May the force be with you.*" This implies that the force is not necessarily with us all the time. In terms of Reiki I would say, "*Remember the force is always with you.*" The difference between these two phrases effectively represents a fundamental difference between Western Reiki for Westerners and Reiki for Japanese. We are connected with source all the time - this is the important message Japanese culture passes on in relation to Reiki.

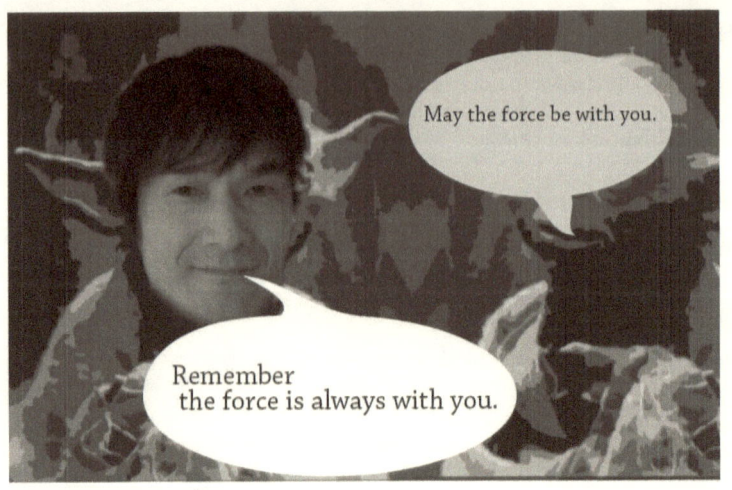

## Shinto

*Ko-shinto* (古神道 ancient Shinto) holds a very important concept called *Ichirei Shikon* (一霊四魂 one spirit, four souls). All matter and organisms, including humans, are born as spirits branched off from the large source. These spirits, once branched are called *Ichirei* (一霊 one spirit). Each

Ichirei may be larger or smaller, but every living thing is derived from source energy and has Ichirei. As such, Koshinto has no idols because we are fully surrounded with its Ichirei. All living things are inherently sacred beings. Humans are said to hold particularly large Ichirei and are thereby capable of performing amazing things depending on

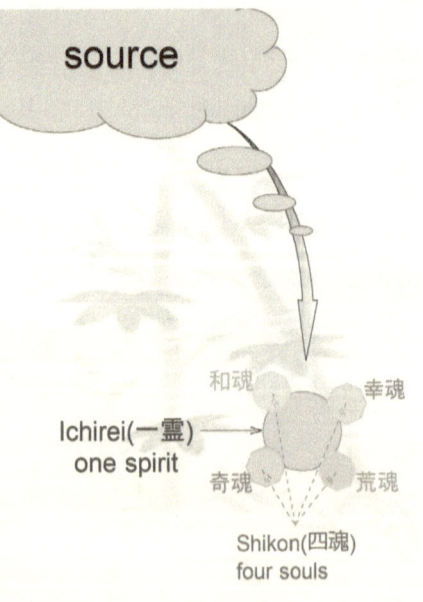

their level of spiritual discipline.

*Shikon* (四魂 four souls) are said to arise around the Ichirei. They serve the function of interfacing with the real world physically, intellectually, emotionally and spiritually. If you are interested in learning more about this, I recommend reading Motohisa Yamakage's, *The Essence of Shinto* (ISBN: 1568364377).

Therefore, each one of us has a core Ichirei that branched from the source, and thus inherently possesses a wonderful power. Of course, not all living beings fully exert this power of Ichirei. Some may develop an evil mentality while living in this secular world. However, in Shinto one can start over again. Through catharsis, re-discipline, or a purification ceremony called Misogi, one can start afresh by cleansing one's mind (Shikon - the four souls) or one can reform, despite past wrongdoings.

This new start is possible because there is a core Ichirei (one spirit) at our center, untouched by the secular world experience. How wonderful it is to be able to re-start life from scratch without going to hell as believed in the Bible or Buddhism!

Given that all living things have Ichirei (a spirit branched from the source), all living things must have Reiki flow.

## Language
The Japanese language contains a unique element rarely found in other

languages. Although Japanese people do not often recognize this notable characteristic, it presents a major challenge to non-Japanese who try to learn the Japanese language. It is connected to the use of transitive and intransitive verbs.

In English, one must clearly define who did what. In Japanese, this is not necessary. The language reflects this and rather than having subjects explicitly spoken, the verb ending is what defines whether someone had a direct hand in the action or it just happened.

As you can see in the example below, changing a few letters, but with the same word order, switches transitive and intransitive modes in Japanese. By doing this, the subject and object are also changed. Intransitive expressions are easily accommodated in the ambiguity of the Japanese language.

For example:

The verb - 離す to release

Transitive: 矢を離す (*Ya wo hana-su*) = I release an arrow.

Intransitive: 矢が離れる (*Ya ga hana-reru*) = The release of an arrow happens.

In Kyudo (Japanese archery), a Western student of Japanese would probably assume that the release of an arrow would use the verb 離す hana-su, which is to consciously release something, as in the example above. However, in Japan a Kyudo practitioner uses the verb 離れる hana-reru, which essentially means, 'the release of an arrow happens,' implying it happens unconsciously, as a natural result, in a natural flow.

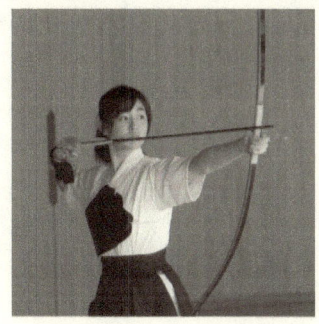

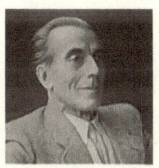

Eugen Herrigel, the author of *Zen in the Art of Archery*, learned Kyudo in the late Taisho era in Japan. In this book he describes how he struggled to understand why the release of an arrow is not 'hana-su' for a long time. He questioned, "If *I* am releasing an arrow, why it is called 'hana-reru'?" It is hard to understand for Westerners.

This applies to Reiki in exactly the same way. I have Reiki coming out of my hand uses the verb 出る deru, but why shouldn't I use 出す dasu for, I draw it out, because I am the one doing the Reiki? I hope, by now, you know the answer to this! It is the same as the release of an arrow in Kyudo.

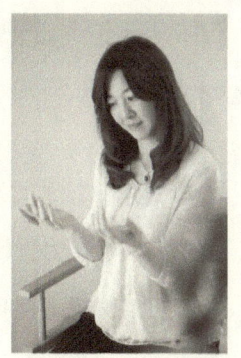

The perception that things happen or are naturally there (being) has been passed on from ancient times as a matter of common sense in Japan and is therefore reflected in the language. To the Western mind, intransitivized expressions tend to be perceived negatively as an evasion of responsibility. In Japan however, such ambiguity is a matter of everyday practice and the

215

language used is therefore formed in this way. Even before language, the Japanese thinking pattern or flow of thought is formed in such a way that subjects are irrelevant. The structure of the Japanese language reflects the structure of their thinking, and the thinking in Japan reflects nature, where things happen spontaneously.

Likewise, Reiki takes no subjects. No one knows where Reiki comes from, it just spontaneously comes out without intention - how typical for something from Japan! Things happen naturally, without intention, this is the essence of Reiki. There is no need to intend to send, intend to draw out or intend to heal someone. As long as we remain in a natural state, Reiki will travel and take effect without intention. For Westerners, who are less likely to consider that things happen naturally, Reiki would be hard to grasp, hard to recognize, or remain unrecognized. Hence Reiki simply could not have been born out of Western culture, it could only have been discovered in Japan, where the natural is allowed to happen.

**Nature teaches us the true Reiki characteristics**
Once again, *in Reiki there is no need to:*
- imagine something
- recite anything
- strain ourselves
- set a clear intention, or
- get connected with something

Instead, all we need do is relax, release the tension in our body and Reiki comes out spontaneously. When we abandon specific intentions, and enter a natural state, Reiki comes out in its purest form.

*By 'natural state' I mean:*

- not trying to heal someone
- leaving it to the person and his or her body
- not straining yourself
- not worrying whether it will work
- not trying too hard, and
- not trying to send anything

The natural state is akin to, 'leaving the self to itself'. It is even close to *iikagen*, which translates as 'being sloppy' or 'being irresponsible'. In English this is only negative, but in Japanese it can also be used positively. Reiki lies in this realm of vagueness, of intransitive verbs. In Reiki, we are indeed not responsible for healing, we are allowing things to happen naturally. We do not 'cure' the other person, they are 'cured' through the natural healing power in their own body.

Nature does not try to give Reiki to others, it does not worry about how powerful it is or isn't and it does not try to become more powerful, yet nature is healing. Nature is simply 'being' and as such, is demonstrating the most powerful use of Reiki.

## Japanese culture today

2,000 years of the Japanese appreciation of *awe before nature* and the concept of '*letting it be*', is what allowed the miracle of Reiki energy to be discovered by Usui in 1922. The 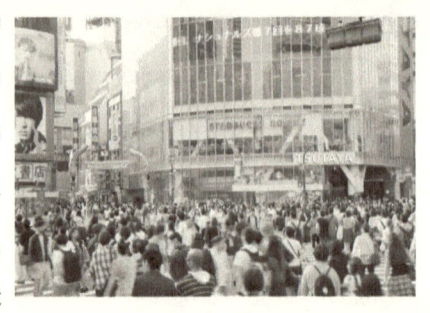 globalization of Japan today, while beneficial in some areas, is threatening that culture. Reiki began its journey from Japan as a deep, integral part of that culture, yet it soon became diluted and many of the gifts it held got lost along the way.

I believe the traditional Japanese perspective on life is vital to the world at large, both in terms of human spiritual cultivation and the survival of the natural world. For this reason, it is the responsibility of Japanese to learn more about their culture so that they can accurately convey it to the outside world.

## Afterword

I always disliked history classes at school and was not good at the subject. It was therefore entirely unexpected that I should end up writing something on history. I became interested in the history of Reiki when I first learned Western Reiki. After the seminar, I felt somehow frustrated, it was as though something was stuck in my throat. I wondered what had been going on when Reiki was established.

My feeling changed when I read the books by Frank Arjava Petter and attended the Jikiden Reiki seminars. These gave me answers to some extent and my frustration diminished somewhat. After that, Takashi Terashima, a shihan of Jikiden Reiki, taught me about Reijutsu-ka and I began to study literature on them. I wrote more and more about the Reiki history I was discovering on my website and studied the history in even greater depth while I was writing my first book.

My awareness definitively changed when I started teaching Jikiden Reiki to foreign students. This made me realize how little I still knew and understood of the Reiki history. Moreover I realized most Japanese people, including myself, do not understand Japan and its culture. However, to my surprise, I found that many foreign people are genuinely interested in Japanese culture. This produced an emotional conflict in me that caused me to write this book.

Some parts of my manuscript are written in great detail and some are brief. Please forgive such irregularity. This book is like my research notes. I hope it helps your daily Reiki practice.

## Acknowledgements

I would like to thank Keiko Moriyama and Ikuko Hirota for translating the Japanese manuscript into English. A special thanks goes to Amanda Jayne who transformed the English manuscript making it far more concise and comprehensible. The editing work with Amanda made my thought deeper and clearer and this book more appealing to Western readers. I am also very grateful to the Hungarian students who have given me various valuable insights.

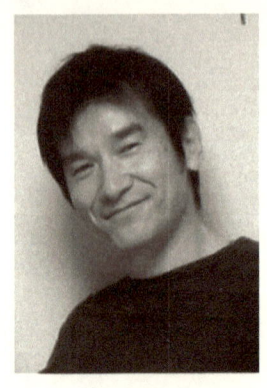

**Masaki Nishina** was born and raised in Tokyo. He used to work in the academic field, unrelated to any therapies. He studied Physics as an undergraduate, engaging in a particle experiment using the world's largest accelerator in his graduate year at Fermi National Accelerator Laboratory in the US. After earning his Ph.D, he turned to Astronomy and began studying clusters of galaxies and observational cosmology, developing the world's biggest wide-field cameras, first as an assistant at the National Astronomical Observatory in Tokyo, then as an associate professor at the Institute for Cosmic Ray Research, University of Tokyo.

Masaki first learned Western Reiki in 2000 and started to work as a therapist and teacher in 2003. Subsequently, he became an aromatherapist certified by the UK ITEC and studied psychological counseling. He learned Jikiden Reiki in 2005 and became dai-shihan in 2010. So far he has taught more than 2,000 Western Reiki students and a few hundred Jikiden Reiki students.

Masaki enjoys Sado and Kyudo as well as Japanese ceramic art and wearing Japanese kimono. He eats meats, drinks coffee and enjoys bourbon and gin as a healthy part of his life, too.